# Cultural Safety in Trauma-Informed Practice from a First Nations Perspective

# Cultural Safety in Trauma-Informed Practice from a First Nations Perspective

## Billabongs of Knowledge

Nicole Tujague • Kelleigh Ryan

Co-design Weaver, Researcher and Editor
Kath Fisher

palgrave
macmillan

Nicole Tujague
Gnibi School of Indigenous Peoples
Southern Cross University
Bilinga, QLD, Australia

Kelleigh Ryan
The Seedling Group
Gold Coast, QLD, Australia

ISBN 978-3-031-13137-0 ISBN 978-3-031-13138-7 (eBook)
https://doi.org/10.1007/978-3-031-13138-7



This Palgrave Macmillan imprint is published by the registered company Springer Nature Switzerland AG.
The registered company address is: Gewerbestrasse 11, 6330 Cham, Switzerland

*Dedication*

*This book is dedicated to our mother, Elaine Dell O'Connor, whose Aboriginal and South Sea Island blood flows in our veins and who re-joined our ancestors during the writing of this book.*

*We also dedicate this book to all the Aboriginal and Torres Strait Islander Peoples of Australia, who have had the strength to survive the ongoing trauma they have endured from the first days of colonisation of our Countries and Nations in 1788 to the present day.*

*We trust that sharing this knowledge from our own perspective will shine light on those strengths.*

# Foreword

It is my great pleasure to write the foreword for *Billabongs of Knowledge*. This book is a unique resource, written by Aboriginal professionals for Aboriginal professionals and the community. Nicole Tujague and Kelleigh Ryan have written this book from the wealth of their collective experience in healing and wellbeing and importantly from an Indigenous perspective.

The intention was to design a resource that is easily accessible and that would benefit anyone who needs to understand what to consider in terms of culture and the effects of trauma for Aboriginal and Torres Strait Islander people. The book provides practical support with actionable information and detailed explanations of wellbeing concepts. This is a valuable resource for both Aboriginal and Torres Strait Islander and non-Indigenous practitioners and gives non-Indigenous practitioners a unique opportunity to gain insight into and hear Indigenous voices.

The authors have considerable experience and training in psychology and educational support and saw the dire need for a trauma-informed approach and developed training programs for this. The book is a resource for the training program but also has general applicability and is appropriate for those working in a broad range of health and social science disciplines. Readers will find this Indigenous lens on trauma and healing a significant departure from the majority of texts available in these fields, which are written predominantly by non-Indigenous authors. Indigenous viewpoints and lived experiences make this book a unique resource that engages the reader in understanding when you listen to Aboriginal and Torres Strait Islander stories in our own words, it makes sense and connects deeply with our own experiences.

Kelleigh based the training program and book on what she saw in her psychology practice with Aboriginal and Torres Strait Islander clients. Taking the best from both worlds, she found that the medical approach of focusing on symptoms lacked understanding of the trauma response system and how it plays out in relationships and behaviours. She knew that the reason for this lack of understanding is based on the fundamental difference between an individualistic non-Indigenous worldview, and a collectivist Aboriginal or Torres Strait Islander cultural worldview. Hence, the training and book values, respects and seeks to strengthen Indigenous knowledges while also using relevant concepts that were appropriate from Western psychology. This knowledge is a fusion of the best scientific and cultural knowledges research and is well informed by the latest research.

I have been honoured to witness a period of change where the terrible impacts of colonisation on our people have been recognised, where the limitations and inappropriateness of Western concepts for our wellbeing have been challenged and the need to have our own knowledges and voice is acknowledged. This is an exciting moment in history as Indigenous knowledges and decolonising research methodologies that will benefit mental health and wellbeing are recognised. *Billabongs of Knowledge* is a manifestation of that transformative change in mental health and wellbeing. It centres Indigenous knowledges and experience but also includes the best of Western knowledge. The empowering process of learning is part of a healing journey for all Australians.

I highly commend this book to all who work in this important area.

Professor Pat Dudgeon

Centre for Best Practice in Aboriginal and Torres
Strait Islander Suicide Prevention, UWA, Perth, WA, Australia
Transforming Indigenous Mental Health and Wellbeing
Million Minds Research Grant, UWA, Perth, WA, Australia
Telethon Institute for Child Health Research, University of
Canberra, Canberra, Australia
Bilya Marlee School of Indigenous Studies, The University of
Western Australia, Perth, WA, Australia

# Preface

We decided to write this book in response to many requests from Aboriginal and Torres Strait Islander participants and Elders who attended our Indigenous-led training programs. Our training programs are very participatory, culturally safe and crammed full of information. Many people told us it would be great to have a book that they could dip into and remind themselves of some of the ideas, practices and useful tips that came up during the workshops and webinars. We thought a book like this would also be helpful for non-Indigenous students, practitioners and educators to witness how First Nations Peoples talk to each other about the issues that affect them. It is very rare to find a book that speaks about the complexities of trauma from a First Nations perspective, in an accessible Australian Indigenous voice. We think this is a book whose time has come.

We would like to acknowledge the support, encouragement and love of our families throughout this journey. Despite losing Mum during the writing of this book we welcomed a new addition to the family, Tanna Arthur Ryan who we hope will live in a world that is freer and more just for First Nations Peoples.

We have drawn on the expertise of many generous people through the writing of this book, including Psychologist Helen Sheehy. Thank you for our robust discussions on polyvagal theory and privileging Indigenous voices.

We would particularly like to thank our sister and Speech Pathologist, Riley O'Connor-Horrill who spent many weeks editing and copyrighting with us, to minimise the risk of anything written in this book being weaponised against First Nations Peoples.

We acknowledge all the people who have attended our training and given back to us more than we can say. Your stories, your humour, your generosity and feedback have been a source of inspiration for this work we do.

Finally, we acknowledge the resilience and beauty of all First Nations Peoples ….

Nicole Tujague<br>Kelleigh Ryan

# Respect for Cultural Protocols

We acknowledge that out of respect for the many different protocols around death and grief and respect for First Nations Peoples, we ask you to be aware that throughout this book there may be photos and names mentioned of people who have passed away.

All stories that are shared about clients are done so with their permissions, and their names, genders and places have been changed to protect their privacy.

# Contents

# About the Authors

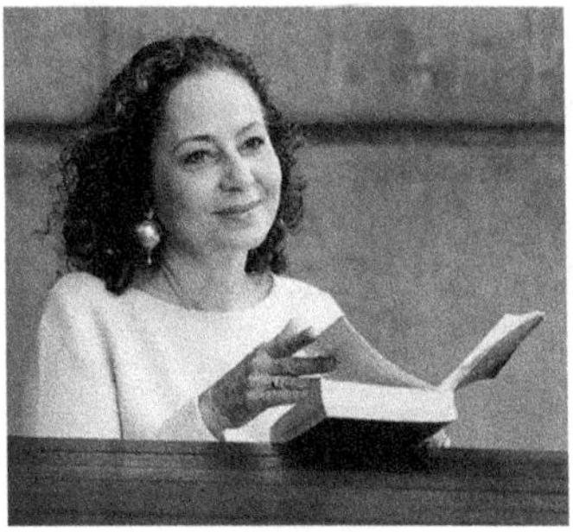

**Nicole Tujague** is one of the two founding directors of The Seedling Group, a consultancy that offers training on cross-cultural safety and trauma-informed practice, particularly in First Nations contexts. She has a Bachelor of Indigenous Studies and is completing a PhD in Indigenous Evaluation Methodology from Australia's Southern Cross University (SCU). She is a board member of the Australian Evaluation Society. Her background includes lecturing at SCU in Indigenous studies and teaching in the vocational education sector and she has many years' experience in face-to-face training and program development. Nicole is passionate about improving the health and well-being of Indigenous Australians through trauma-informed, evidence-based practices and culturally appropriate evaluation.

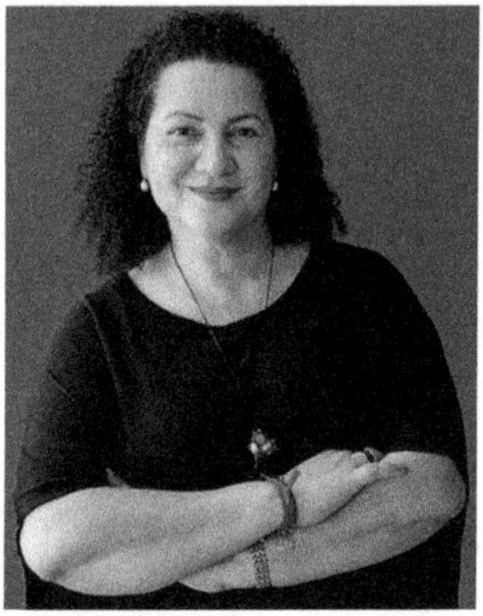

**Kelleigh Ryan** is Director and Consulting Psychologist for The Seedling Group, a Fellow of the Australian Psychological Society and Vice Chair of the Australian Indigenous Psychologists Association. She completed her degree in psychology at Griffith University in Brisbane, Australia. Kelleigh specialises in trauma and social consultancy, which explores change at the individual, family and collective levels and is part of the decolonising psychology movement. She is a fellow of the Australian Psychological Society. Her work has been recognised through a Lifetime Achievement Award from Indigenous Allied Health Australia (IAHA) for supporting Aboriginal and Torres Strait Islander allied health professionals. Kelleigh has also been a supervisor for the staff of *Link-Up* Queensland, an Indigenous organisation that reconnects members of The Stolen Generations who were separated from family and culture by past government policies through forced removal, being fostered, adopted or raised in institutions.

## Co-design Weaver, Researcher and Editor

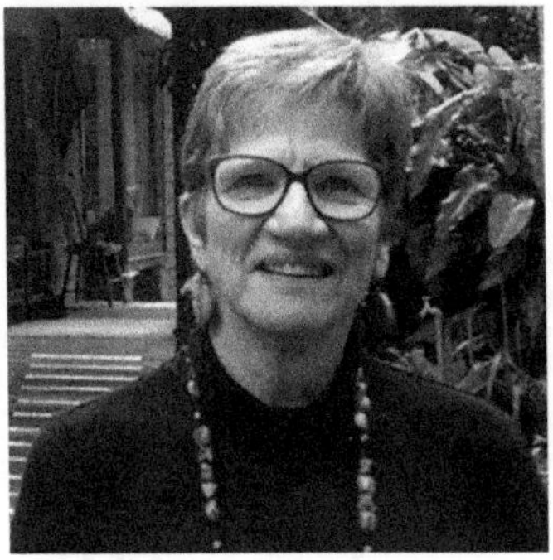

**Kath Fisher** is an experienced teacher, academic mentor, writer and editor. She has had various roles teaching and supporting students in universities and vocational education since the 1970s. Her research interests are in teaching critical self-reflection in the context of experiential and community-engaged learning. Kath has worked at Southern Cross University since 1995, where she is an adjunct fellow in community engagement.

# List of Figures

# 1

# Introducing Billabongs of Knowledge

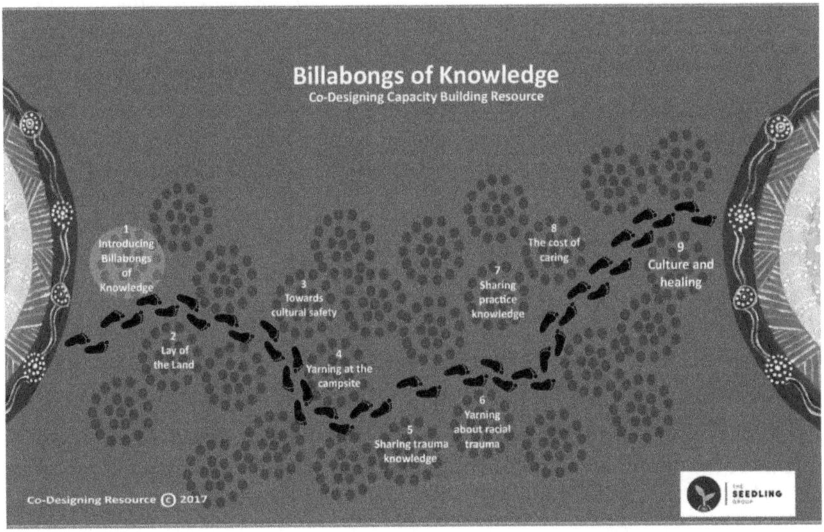



N. Tujague, K. Ryan, *Cultural Safety in Trauma-Informed Practice from a First Nations Perspective*, https://doi.org/10.1007/978-3-031-13138-7_1

## Honouring the Ancestors

Today we stand in footsteps millennia old.
May we acknowledge the traditional owners
Whose cultures and customs have nurtured,
And continue to nurture, this land,
Since men and women
Awoke from the great dream.

We honour the presence of these ancestors
Who reside in the imagination of this land
And whose irrepressible spirituality
Flows through all creation.

*Jonathan Hill, Aboriginal Poet*

*Secondary sources attribute this poem to Aboriginal poet Jonathan Hill, unfortunately we were unable to confirm his authorship through any primary source.*

## Who This Book Is for

This book was written for you, the Indigenous professional working at the grassroots, the student who is preparing to work in this space and for our non-Indigenous allies who work and study alongside us. You may have picked up this book because you, like us, care about the wellbeing of First Nations Peoples and communities and your work is far more than just a job. If you are a student, thank you for having the courage to learn about cultural safety in trauma-informed practice before you enter our communities. We have written this book with care, respect and down to earth practical knowledge about trauma-informed practice. What you will read about is critical to understand because of Australia's stories of colonisation, genocide and displacement of people from Country. The devastating impacts of early colonisation in Australia are just as potent today. These impacts have forged a gap in social and health outcomes between the expectations of the general Australian population and the experience of Australia's First Nations Peoples. We know you will find some useful information that supports your work. We trust it will enhance your understanding of the clinical and cultural implications of the impacts of colonisation on First Nations Peoples across the world. The book is designed to be an addition to your toolkit. Take care of yourself as you work through these pages and keep your mind and heart open as you learn through the lens of First Nations Peoples.

*Nicole and Kelleigh.*

## Who Are We? A Personal Introduction to Us and Our Family

You can read about our professional achievements in the front of this book, but here we share some of our personal story and family connections. While the system of meritocracy wants to see evidence of our qualifications and our achievements that gives us the right to talk in the non-Indigenous world, for Indigenous Peoples it is our cultural understandings, lived experience and family connections that give us the right to speak in our world.

We are sisters and descendants of Australian Aboriginal and South Sea Islander Peoples. Our mother is a descendant of tribal woman Sarah Lloyd of the *Kabi Kabi* people, whose country is in South-Eastern Queensland, Australia. Our great grandfather was among those taken from the Island of Gaua in Vanuatu and brought across to Queensland to work as a slave in the cane fields. We grew up on the Aboriginal and Torres Strait Islander communities of Bamaga, Kowanyama, Woorabinda and Yarrabah in Queensland. Our heritage is one of immense resilience and collective healing borne out of generations of lived experience.

***Nicole:*** *My name is Nicole Tujague and I was born under a tree in Springsure in country Queensland on the lands of the Wadja Wadja/Wadjigal people, where my Dad delivered me. I was extremely privileged to hold Dad's hand when he went to join the ancestors some years ago. I'm a sister, an auntie, a great auntie and the mother of a beautiful son. I'm a co-founder of The Seedling Group with my sister Kelleigh.*

***Kelleigh**: And I'm Kelleigh Ryan. I'm Nicole's sister, the other co-founder of our organisation. I'm a daughter, a mother of two beautiful girls and a nanna. I'm also a psychologist and specialise in trauma and social consultancy, which explores change on the individual, community and collective levels.*

*My first experience of understanding the impact of trauma was when we went to our uncle's funeral while I was doing my undergraduate degree. An old family friend said to me, "I live out here alone because if I decided to kill myself, it would be a long time before anyone found me." When I started to think about the story of their family and history, that was the first time I started to see the impacts of trauma passed down within families.*

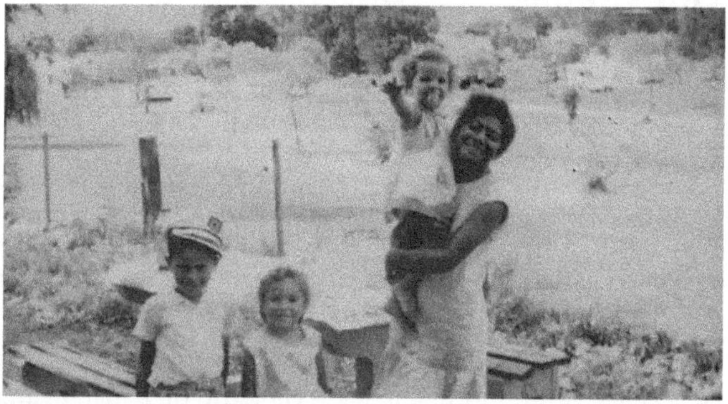

This is one of our favourite family photos, taken by our Dad, of us as kids with our Mum. The little girl in Mum's arms is Kelleigh. The little boy is our brother Chris, the first-born child. Standing next to him is Nicole. Chris is part of The Seedling Group team and does research and men's work for us in Aboriginal and Torres Strait Islander communities. When mum was expecting Chris, she was prescribed Thalidomide, a drug used to treat morning sickness and banned in Australia in 1961 for causing birth defects. We were very lucky, because mum was so sick, she threw up the Thalidomide after she'd taken it; because she didn't digest it, Chris was spared crippling side effects.

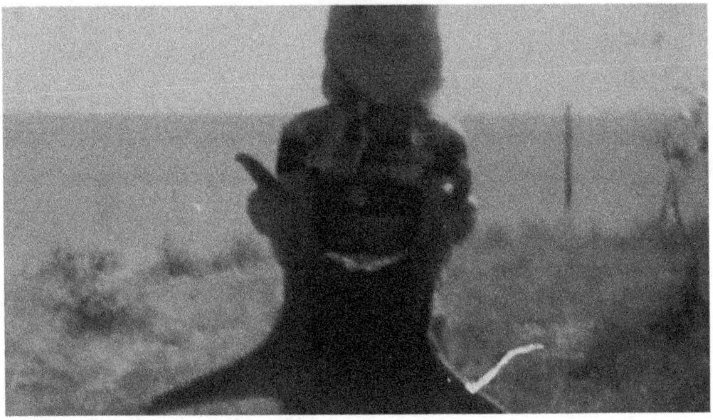

Our little sister Riley was born after the family photo above was taken, but here she is, holding a spectacular starfish up on Cape York when she was little. We find this photo amazing, because starfish this size are rarely seen in this area today. This loss of species is a form of environmental trauma that Aboriginal and Torres Strait Islander Peoples experience at the front line of climate change. Riley is a speech pathologist who works on our content and researches trauma from the perspective of how it affects children's speech, language and communication development.

Another important member of our Seedling Group family is Donna Hensen, who has worked with our team for some years. Donna is a well-known Aboriginal artist, counsellor and art therapist. She drew our Billabongs of Knowledge map and other artworks throughout the book. Donna often attends our trainings to support Aboriginal and Torres Strait Islander participants, as hearing and learning about trauma can be triggering. Donna is a descendant of *Wailwan/Wiradjuri* people of New South Wales and a survivor of the 'Stolen Generations'.

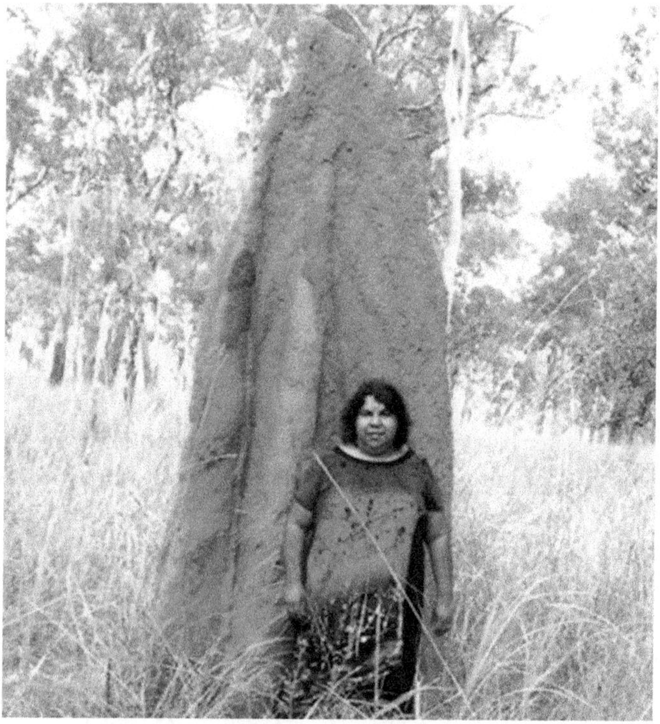

## What Is the Story Behind This Book?

Since before colonisation, the Aboriginal and Torres Strait Islander cultural systems have been holistic, balanced and deeply connected to all things. The systems allowed any shift out of balance in our environment to be noticed and understood so that balance could quickly be restored. While there were still traumas, they were accepted and understood as part of being.

Each of us had different but connected paths that brought us to the point of writing this book:

**Kelleigh:** My path was influenced through my work with Aboriginal and Torres Strait Islander clients in my psychology practice; with The Aboriginal and Torres Strait Islander Healing Foundation; and with the

Royal Commission into Institutional Responses to Child Sexual Abuse. I did a national audit of the skill levels that existed in Aboriginal and Torres Strait Islander organisations that were funded to do the work of supporting victims in relation to the findings of the Royal Commission. I found that almost all Aboriginal and Torres Strait Islander organisations were using strong cultural healing practices. However, Australian Government funding privileged organisations that used mainstream clinical practices, organisations that often did not have relationships with Aboriginal and Torres Strait Islander communities. I was part of the argument posed at the time, that to support Aboriginal and Torres Strait Islander Peoples who were victims of institutional child abuse, we need *both* cultural healing expertise *and* clinical practice expertise.

In designing training for these Aboriginal and Torres Strait Islander organisations we found that many staff were best supported through an intensive, experiential two-day training program, rather than a long-form diploma or certificate course. This is consistent with how knowledge was passed on traditionally: people came together, learnt new skills, practised and applied what they had learned when they returned to their own community settings.

This training was based on what I was seeing in my psychology practice with Aboriginal and Torres Strait Islander clients. I saw that the medical approach of focusing on symptoms lacked understanding of the trauma response system and how it plays out in relationships and behaviours. The reason for this lack of understanding is based on the fundamental difference between an individualistic non-Indigenous worldview, and a collectivist Aboriginal or Torres Strait Islander cultural worldview. What you need for evidence in a non-Indigenous worldview already exists in our First Nations worldview. The non-Indigenous scientific method of 'evidence-based practice' is no different from the ancient practice of combining ingredients of known value to achieve an outcome, telling the story so that others can replicate it, modifying the ingredients when or as the situation requires and sharing this knowledge at multi-Nation gatherings.

**Nicole:** My path started with my experience of working in the area of trauma and its impacts when I was manager of student support for students from 91 Indigenous communities, all of whom were staying in different private boarding schools across Australia. My role involved supporting Aboriginal and Torres Strait Islander students and their families and communities around issues of intergenerational trauma, mental health and coping with non-Indigenous environments. I saw how many Aboriginal and Torres Strait Islander students experienced racism and punitive measures at the hands of educators because of the non-Indigenous educators' lack of knowledge about the ways trauma is lived out. I launched a peer support program for student support staff to ensure they received appropriate psychological supervision while they were working with Aboriginal and Torres Strait Islander students and their families.

This experience ultimately led me to teach Indigenous health at university. Through this teaching experience, I realised that when we talk about Aboriginal and Torres Strait Islander cultures and health issues, we really need to understand trauma and include it in the curriculum. The students I was teaching, who were studying to be podiatrists, nurses, speech pathologists and other allied health practitioners, weren't getting any information about trauma through their curriculum. It seemed obvious to me that understanding trauma is vital for these students, because once you learn about trauma in a culturally safe way, you can understand not only what's happening to people's bodies, but also what's happening in their families and communities. This knowledge can then inform diagnosis and care or treatment plans.

As we had each been working in different areas of Indigenous social and emotional wellbeing, we realised that what our experiences had in common was that the psychological trauma that began with colonisation wasn't getting the attention it deserved. It was clearly the 'elephant in the room'.

While each of us has our own distinctive skill set, the common thread is that we are family. We have always walked in both the Indigenous and non-Indigenous worlds, which is a gift as well as a challenge. Both our experiences combined to light the fire of our desire to share knowledge about trauma in an Aboriginal way, using *our* way of speaking, privileging *our* cultural ways of knowing, being and doing, telling *our* stories, recognising *our* strengths in the way we have survived and continue to learn. It felt like the ancestors were speaking to us; spirit put us in places we would not usually find ourselves, which made things happen; it was

Country saying *this is important.* It was coming from people's pain and witnessing their empowerment when they began to understand more about trauma. Not sharing this knowledge would be to continue the injustice.

Writing the book has been a weaving process of experiences, what we've learnt along the way, what community has told us, what non-Indigenous science tells us and how we navigate and walk in both worlds.

## How Is This Book Different?

The knowledge sharing in this book has been an Indigenous-led process. Our intention was to design a resource that is easily accessible. It will benefit anyone who needs to understand what to consider in terms of culture and the effects of trauma for First Nations' Peoples. Aboriginal and Torres Strait Islander Peoples who have attended our cultural safety in trauma-informed practice training in community or through our webinars, will find this book provides practical support with actionable information and fuller explanations of concepts introduced in the training.

We speak as Australian Aboriginal authors, in our Aboriginal way of talking, from our own experience and within an Indigenous Knowledge framework of healing practice. When we each speak from our individual experiences, stories or perspectives, our individual voices will be in *italics* to distinguish them from our combined 'training' way of delivering information. We trust this will give all our readers a deeper sense of how things are for us as Indigenous Peoples, we who have been dealing with the impact of complex trauma since the time of early colonisation.

The book is also a textbook for students who are likely to work with First Nations' Peoples within a broad range of health and social science disciplines. Students will find the Indigenous lens on trauma and healing a significant departure from the majority of texts available in these fields, which are written predominantly by non-Indigenous authors. There is much more to understand when you listen to Aboriginal and Torres Strait Islander stories in our own words.

For university students and practitioners interested in evidence-based research papers, we include more in-depth literature sections in some chapters, titled "Want to know more about …?", which review relevant academic literature about particular topics and offer a guide to further reading at the end of each chapter. Whether you are a student, a practitioner or community member, Indigenous or non-Indigenous, you will find a different style and approach from what you would be used to seeing in standard textbooks and hear a different voice from that which is usually privileged.

## Why 'Billabongs of Knowledge'?

We decided to use the metaphor of the 'billabong' for our training because for some Aboriginal people billabongs have a special cultural meaning. First Nations Peoples have used stories and metaphors for generations to pass down knowledge. According to some sources, the word 'billabong' is derived from the *Wiradjuri*[1] word *bilabang*: *bila* means 'river' and *bang* means 'continuing in time or space'. Billabongs are the remnant waterholes left after a meandering river system has been forced to go in a more direct line to its destination. Sometimes even when the billabongs dry up, there's still water underneath that comes back up again when there's rain. When the river floods, the water in the billabong flows again as it connects with the main river. Because of this, the water stays fresh and supports an abundance of life. Billabongs were an important source of water and food for Aboriginal Peoples because they remain for long periods during the dry season.

We developed the Billabongs of Knowledge concept very early in our teaching and training. The idea was that when you're ready to drink from a certain billabong, it's only then that you can take in the knowledge.

The other reason we wanted to use billabongs as the central metaphor for our training is that it represents the way colonisation changed the landscape for our people. First Nations cultures have always been

[1] The *Wiradjuri* Aboriginal Nation is situated in a large area in south western New South Wales, inland from Sydney.

collective, in balance with nature. When colonisation came along, often rivers were manipulated to follow planned routes. They were no longer living in balance with nature. The rivers were forced to take a more direct path, not a winding or meandering route. But what we know is that those billabongs, while they may dry up on the surface, water (knowledge) remains below. It's about reflecting on what is very important culturally, understanding that a strong healing knowledge still lies there, sometimes visible, sometimes just beneath the dry riverbed. You only need to be shown how to dig down to find this knowledge.

## How Are the Chapters in the Book Structured?

Each chapter represents a different billabong along the journey of knowledge-sharing about cultural safety in trauma-informed practice, a journey that takes us from understanding to healing. Each chapter begins with the map that highlights the billabong that represents where we are along the journey. Each billabong can also stand alone. The journey is not linear. It meanders like the river. You can make a choice about how long you want to sit at one of the billabongs on the journey and what knowledge you're ready to take with you.

As well as highlighting where we are on the Billabongs of Knowledge Map, we start each chapter with an 'Acknowledgement of Country'. This is a practice increasingly embraced in Australia, that acknowledges the land (or Country) on which people meet or gather for a purpose, and as importantly, the traditional custodians and Elders of that land. We encourage you to incorporate this practice into your gatherings, wherever they may be held. This is because wherever you are in Australia, remember you are on Aboriginal land. Recognise that sovereignty of this land was never ceded. There was never a treaty, as there was in New Zealand and other countries.

We begin each chapter with a 'check-in', where you check how you are feeling and where you feel it in your body. This is designed to make you aware of your mental and physical state so that you can recognise when or if that changes as you experience the knowledge sharing at each billabong. We offer examples of grounding exercises, or 'somatic experiencing tools', to help you take care of yourself while you learn with an open mind. We have designed these exercises in a way that may be useful to you as you read this book, to incorporate into your life, or that you may offer to or share with your clients. At the end of each chapter, we ask you to 'check-out' and offer reflective questions designed to deepen your understanding as you go through your learning journey.

## About Each Chapter

### Chapter 2: The Lay of the Land

At this billabong we yarn about some of the ways we share knowledge and what is important to consider when working with First Nations Peoples in Australia. We the authors, belong to one of many mobs who are First Nations Australians, our voices are one of many voices. Throughout the book we aim to privilege Indigenous voices and perspectives while drawing on both cultural and mainstream knowledge systems. Our style of sharing knowledge is through yarning and sharing stories, like we would be sharing if we were sitting at the billabong with you. We shy away from the deficit language usually used to describe our mobs and focus on what has healed us and kept us strong. We are careful to keep you the reader safe, so there are checking in, checking out and grounding and self-reflection protocols to explore. Billabong 2 is about how we as Aboriginal knowledge sharers will be yarning with you at the billabongs in this book.

### Chapter 3: The Journey Towards Cultural Safety: Cultural Safety in Trauma-Informed Practice from an Indigenous Perspective

This billabong is where we sit and yarn about cultural safety and what it means for us as First Nations Peoples. We also examine how cultural safety is difficult to achieve without understanding trauma. This is where we talk about how trauma and cultural safety impacts us on every level from our cells and body systems to our families, communities and the environment. These levels are all independent yet interdependent, they are related in complex ways, and healing of all of these parts is a holistic concept. To move along the continuum of cultural safety, we begin to look at Indigenous values and ways of being.

## Chapter 4: Yarning at the Campsite: Understanding Trauma

At this billabong, we discuss what this thing called trauma is and why it is so important to know about when working with First Nations Peoples. It is incredibly liberating to understand how trauma affects the brain and the body and how our responses of befriend, fight, flee and freeze are ways that our bodies keep us safe. The ACE study is explored at this billabong as it has important implications for us as First Nations Peoples, as does what we know about how attachment theory is different for us, and how polyvagal theory can tell us more about how we respond to trauma.

## Chapter 5: Sharing Trauma Knowledge: Types of Trauma

At this billabong we set up camp and dig down into more detail about the different types of trauma that affect us as human beings, and how for colonised peoples that trauma can be multi-layered and complex to recognise and heal from. Some of the traumas such as institutional trauma, intergenerational trauma and historical trauma as well as developmental trauma, can be triggering to read about if you have a trauma story yourself, so take care when sitting at this billabong.

## Chapter 6: Yarning about Racial Trauma

At Billabong 6 we yarn about racial trauma and the impact it has on us as First Nations Peoples. We notice how racism can be obvious and socially unacceptable but how it also hides in policies and procedures that erode our social and emotional wellbeing. Recognising and naming different ways that racism shows up in every day life can be empowering as we get better at calling it out and understanding why it makes us, the perpetrator and the receiver, unwell. Racism leads to harmful practices such as stereotyping and dehumanising which perpetuates colonising acts. At this billabong, allies can reflect upon how to avoid being involved in covert racial practices. We discuss why meritocracy is the language of shame and how to recognise the cultural load we often find ourselves carrying.

## Chapter 7: Sharing Practice Knowledge

Now that we have been thinking about trauma and the many ways it affects our lives, at this billabong we look at different models and frameworks that we can use to move towards cultural safety in trauma-informed practice. We won't always know our client's trauma story, so working in a culturally safe and trauma-informed way ensures that we create a space where we do no further harm and promote healing. We recognise at this billabong collective cultures and holistic ways of healing as well as mainstream models useful to have in your toolkit.

## Chapter 8: Compassion Fatigue, Vicarious Trauma and Self-care

At this billabong we yarn about what happens when we work with those who have a trauma story and how we can keep ourselves safe. Lots of different terms are used to describe this 'secondary' trauma and we investigate the differences and how they impact us. Remember, it is normal for your body to react on many levels to others' trauma stories, it's not *if* you will react, but noticing *when* your body reacts. For many of us it is the price we pay for being exposed to *'truth telling'* and this billabong helps us understand the importance of working safely, practicing self-care and taking the opportunity to replenish. With this knowledge, we can work towards building a sustainable work life.

## Chapter 9: Culture and Healing

This yarning session takes a little bit of a winding road, as yarns often do. This is a new story, the story of healing. We look at the psychology of culture and what *healing*-informed practice (different to *trauma*-informed practice) looks like. We discuss why this is important, and how and why we privilege Indigenous Knowledges and Indigenous voices. While for many Aboriginal and Torres Strait Islander Peoples culture is still strong and thrives despite colonisation, for others this is not the case. We talk about how we're starting to reconnect the pieces of culture that were fractured by colonisation. We offer examples of cultural practices in Aboriginal and Torres Strait Islander cultures that promote healing. These include things like language, connection to Country, linking up families, yarning, *dadirri* (deep listening), rituals and ceremonies.

# 2

# The Lay of the Land

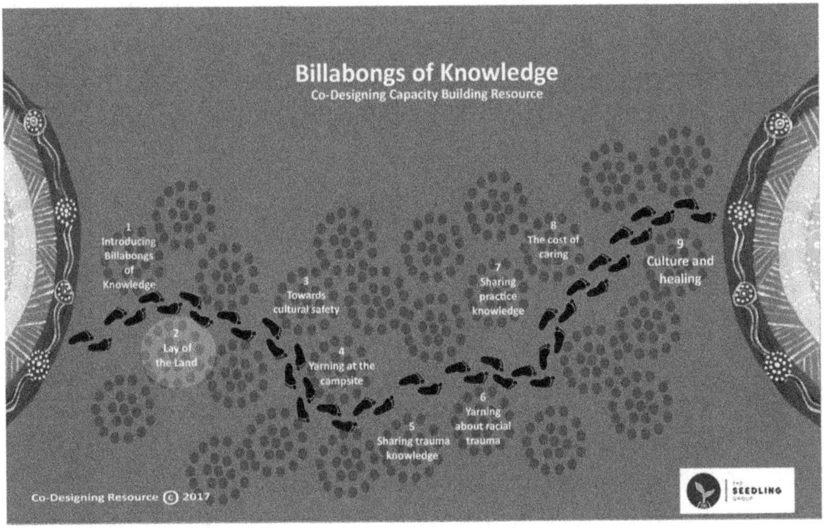


We acknowledge the traditional custodians of the lands on which we meet. We thank them for their beautiful custodianship and for saving our stories and songlines to pass on to our young people. We pay our respects to Elders, past, present, and emerging, understanding this always was and always will be Aboriginal land.



N. Tujague, K. Ryan, *Cultural Safety in Trauma-Informed Practice from a First Nations Perspective*, https://doi.org/10.1007/978-3-031-13138-7_2

## Introduction

At this billabong we begin with a brief introduction to the diversity of Aboriginal and Torres Strait Islander Nations across Australia. We outline the culture of the book and the principles that underpin our practice: how we privilege Indigenous perspectives, work across Indigenous and mainstream knowledge systems and use an Indigenous storytelling (yarning) approach that is underpinned by strengths-based rather than deficit-based understandings of trauma. We offer a rationale for the types of activities we use throughout the book: checking-in and checking-out, grounding exercises and self-reflection and we touch on what it means to understand your 'knowledge system'. We introduce you to the approach to healing that is most appropriate for Aboriginal and Torres Strait Islander peoples, based on holistic understandings of social and emotional wellbeing informed by cultural wisdom and practices.

## Acknowledging Australia's First Nations Peoples

This QR code and link will take you to a map which shows the many different Language groups that make up Aboriginal and Torres Strait Islander Australia (Fig. 2.1). According to AIATSIS (Australian Institute of Aboriginal and Torres Strait Islander Studies), Australia has over 250 Indigenous languages, with more than 800 dialects spoken. Their website defines languages as "living things that connect people to Country, culture and Ancestors".[1] The AIATSIS website and that of The Healing Foundation[2] are both excellent resources to help you grow your knowledge about Indigenous cultures in Australia and our history of colonisation.

We still recognise those different Nations that represent Aboriginal and Torres Strait Islander Peoples. When we meet another Aboriginal person, often we will say, "who's your mob" and that's our way of saying,

[1] https://aiatsis.gov.au/explore/living-languages

[2] https://healingfoundation.org.au/

**Fig. 2.1** Link to AIATSIS map of Indigenous Australia (https://aiatsis.gov.au/explore/map-indigenous-australia)

"where are you from?" Australia has a very complex history of colonisation, specifically the ongoing impact of removals and people being forced on to different places, often far away from their traditional lands. If one of us meets someone from Cherbourg, we know we are possibly related to someone that they're related to. While Cherbourg is on the traditional lands of the *Wakka Wakka* people, a mission was established there in 1899 and many people were sent there when they were forcibly moved off their own lands. A lot of our people, *Kabi Kabi* people, were moved to Cherbourg and many died in the cold winters there. Making those connections is this contextual and traditional thing we do all the time as Aboriginal and Torres Strait Islander Peoples. This is an important part of practising our living history, through reconnecting storylines. It tells the storyline of connection, of mob and place and relationship.

If you're reading this book as a First Nations person from somewhere else in the world, you will have your own story about belonging and how you contextually situate yourself. The most important thing about this map is to remember that despite all the skyscrapers and buildings and concrete that are part of our Australian landscape today, we are still on Aboriginal land… our refrain is: '*always was, always will be Aboriginal land*'.

For the purposes of comparison, we sometimes superimpose Europe over the top of the Indigenous Australian map, just to give you an idea of how many Nations we are looking at here. Often non-Indigenous people think that if you're Aboriginal, you just belong to this great big group and that your skills or your Aboriginal knowledge are transferable. On one level that's true, but the peoples of each Nation have their own lore, their own storylines, their own ways of knowing, being and doing. For example, for people from our Nation, eating saltwater fish feels very nourishing because we are saltwater people. It is in our DNA to have enzymes that digest food from the salt water and our lungs are able to breathe the moist salty air. Embedded in our genes are eons of social and emotional wellbeing grounded in living near, eating from, relaxing and finding balance in the sounds, smells and sights of being one with the saltwater life. But people from the desert, for example, have different enzymes; their wellbeing is grounded in the dry, desert air and the foods found in that part of the country.

To be culturally safe or to respect the culture of the land where you are visiting, you need to be aware of that. This is why we start each training, each webinar, each chapter of this book, with an acknowledgement that we are standing on or speaking from someone else's land and offer our respects to Elders, past, present and emerging.

**Activity 2.1 Who am I?**

Checking in to Country: If you are in Australia, whose country are you standing on? If you are not in Australia, whose ancestral country are you standing on? Who are the First Nations custodians of the land you are on now? If you don't know, you can find out by checking on the Internet, or talking to your local Aboriginal Medical Service or Land Council.

## The Culture of the Book

The culture of this book is to share, to heal, and to deconstruct and reconstruct knowledge. In the same way that Salzman (2018) talks about culture being a map of how to live your life, the culture of the book is a roadmap of how the process of coming to an understanding of trauma actually works in practice. The following four elements describe how we put the culture of the book into practice.

## We Privilege an Indigenous Perspective

As we deliver our training through an Indigenous and trauma-informed lens, this book is also written from that point of view. We are used to hearing information from a Western, non-Indigenous perspective, which operates within a system that does not speak to our Indigenous stories. Knowledge is power as it gives choice and helps people find better ways to navigate their lives. While trauma-informed practice training itself is powerful, when it's done in a culturally safe way from an Indigenous perspective, it's even more so. We maintain that it is our *right* to practice with our own ways of knowing, being and doing. We also include images, stories, cartoons, symbols, diagrams and links to short videos, consistent with the 'Aboriginal *8-ways of learning*' Aboriginal pedagogy (Yunkaporta & Kirby, 2011; Yunkaporta & McGinty, 2009) that is expressed as "eight interconnected pedagogies involving narrative-driven learning, visualised learning processes, hands-on/reflective techniques, use of symbols/metaphors, land-based learning, indirect/synergistic logic, modelled/scaffolded genre mastery, and connectedness to community."[3]

## We Take a Strengths-Based Approach

There's an African proverb that Kelleigh likes that's very appropriate for us: "Until the story of the hunt is told by the lion, the hunter will always be glorified." We all know that the colonisers get to tell the story. They have no interest in telling our stories from a strengths-based point of view. Our strengths can be found in many places like spirit, Dreaming stories, connection to language and songlines (Neale & Kelly, 2020). These strengths are powerful, passed down to us from our ancestors, in our DNA and our customs. When we move into that whole story of trauma from a strengths-based perspective, we look for the strength that allowed us to still be here today. We distinguish between a 'coping behaviour' that you may have developed in response to trauma (like

[3] Source: 8ways.online.

disassociating to the avoid feeling the pain) and the strength that fuelled the choice you made in that moment of threat (like keeping your family together and safe).

## We Emphasise Self-Care Throughout the Journey

Throughout this book we talk about trauma. We know that learning about traumatic events will activate the threat response in any healthy brain and body. While this is normal, if you still carry 'unresolved trauma' or 'deep pain', your mind may still be navigating the world through a heightened threat response and may be more easily activated into a befriend/fight/flight/freeze response. While this is your brain doing the job of keeping you safe, it can bring back traumatic experiences that you or someone in your life may have had. This memory is often referred to as the 'trigger'. Simply put, if there is a memory with enough emotional energy attached to it, your body will respond. This is your body and spirit remembering to keep you safe.

We believe it's important to stay safe when we share knowledge in this way. What we want to emphasise is that the training we offer is not therapy, it is knowledge sharing. And through this knowledge sharing, we hope you will support and take care of yourself. The grounding exercises and the check-in and check-out in each chapter are designed to support your self-care.

## We Take an Aboriginal 'Yarning' Approach to Sharing Knowledge

'Yarning' is a term based on traditional oral methods of communication and storytelling in Aboriginal and Torres Strait Islander cultures. 'Yarning circles' are similar to cultural knowledge-sharing processes present in many Indigenous cultures around the world. For our purposes, we think of each chapter as a separate 'yarn' at the billabong, in which we share knowledge about trauma and trauma-informed practices. Within each yarn, we tell our own stories, the stories of Aboriginal and Torres Strait Islander Peoples across Australia.

For many years non-Indigenous people have been telling the story of Indigenous Peoples. This is why it is important to tell our own stories, Aboriginal and Torres Strait Islander stories, in our training and through this book. It is only recently that we as Aboriginal and Torres Strait Islander Peoples, have started to have a voice in mainstream storytelling. A lot of the stories that are told about us are told by somebody else, and we have been hearing somebody else's story about us for too long. Some have even come to believe those stories about us, and many stories pathologise us as a whole community. When most people in Australia think about Aboriginal and Torres Strait Islander Peoples, they think suicides; they think chronic poor health; they think early age of deaths. This kind of pathologising is a form of racism. These are not *our* stories. Mainstream stories forget to talk about our strengths like our resilience and our successes. This is why it is especially important to take a strengths-based perspective when we talk about Aboriginal and Torres Strait Islander cultures, rather than one that continues to pathologise.

### Want to Know More About Yarning in Aboriginal Culture?

We share knowledge about culturally-safe, trauma-informed practice through storytelling. In Australia, Aboriginal and Torres Strait Islander Peoples often refer to this approach as 'yarning'. As we shall discuss here, there are different types of yarning depending on the context and intention, each having its own principles and protocols.

**The role of storytelling in Indigenous cultures**

Storytelling has been central to all Indigenous cultures since the first humans walked the earth. Stories have been handed down orally over countless generations and 'preserved as a survival tool for the people as a collective treasured experience' (Lawrence & Paige, 2016, p. 64). These oral traditions represent 'a way of connecting to each other's experiences regardless of time, place and culture' (Jackson-Barrett et al., 2015, p. 37). For most Indigenous peoples, including Australian Aboriginal Peoples, stories are not just about human beings but also 'beings such as plants, wildlife, rocks, thunder, water, wind, and sun, which are all considered to be as alive as the breath that carries them from one person to another' (Lawrence & Paige, 2016, p. 65). It's important to keep in mind as you read and connect with the stories that this allows you to engage with an Aboriginal worldview. We use narrative as a way of making connections with people and place, allowing you to come into contact with 'stories of country, connection and identity' (Somerville et al., 2010, p. 96).

**What is Yarning?**

In simple terms, Yarning for Aboriginal and Torres Strait Islander Peoples means having a conversation. But it can occur at many levels, from informal conversations among family and friends, to more formal communications when 'Elders pass on Knowledge to the next generation' (Hughes & Barlo, 2020, p. 355). This is how *Bwgcolman* woman, Lynore K Geia from Palm Island, Queensland, describes Yarning:

> Aboriginal and Torres Strait Island storytelling, what we call yarning, is not a static process; it begins and it progresses, through loud and raucous engagement, to a sudden move into contemplation and silence. Aboriginal yarning is a fluid ongoing process, a moving dialogue interspersed with interjections, interpretations, and additions. The stories remain in our conscious state like a thread hanging, waiting to be picked up again, to be continued, reconstructed, reinforced and once again embedded in our ontology. Yarning almost always contains the threads of Aboriginal and Torres Strait Island history as it moves into the present tense, its parameters within present time [are] filtered through the memories of the past as the two move simultaneously and at points collide and reveal fragments of the future (Geia et al., 2013, p. 15).

Yarning is also a form of storytelling 'that involves both sound and silence', requiring 'embodied deep listening through which stories emerge that create new knowledge and understanding' (Terare & Rawsthorne, 2020, p. 944). Wiradjuri Elder, Uncle Larry Maxwell Towney, describes Yarning as a unique part of Indigenous culture that is linked to spirituality, thus becoming a 'special and powerful way Aboriginal people connect to each other' (Towney, 2005, p. 40). In this way it establishes relationality and determines accountability (Martin, 2008), being both a process and exchange, encompassing elements of respect, protocol and engagement in individuals' relationships with each other (Fredericks et al., 2011, p. 13).

Yuin man Stuart Barlo (2016) made an in-depth study of the Yarning process with his yarns with senior Aboriginal men for his PhD. He describes Yarning as a 'relational methodology for transferring Indigenous knowledge that dates back to the origins of time… within an Indigenous perspective knowledge is a dynamic living entity with the ability to release information in a manner that safeguards its integrity (Barlo et al., 2020, p. 8). In the research process, he identified different layers of yarns, the deepest of which 'required the most formal adherence to its associated protocols and principles. This yarning layer was identified as being traditionally utilised when an Elder imparts specific knowledge, thus requiring the person receiving the knowledge to be very focused and attentive' (Barlo et al., 2020, p. 2).

**Yarning and healing from the trauma of colonisation**

> For the past two hundred years, Aboriginal people's stories about ourselves have been shaped by what others have said about us. When the mainstream culture describes you in negative ways, this dominant narrative becomes highly destructive to individual lives, families and communities ... We believe that healing comes from reclaiming our lost stories, and through telling and re-telling these stories we can develop a stronger sense of identity and belonging... Over time, the talk deepens, life stories are shared, issues are tackled, traditional practices are remembered, and healing and dignity starts to grow (Towney, 2005, pp. 40, 41).

These are the words of Uncle Larry, who worked for many years with Aboriginal men who had lost their sense of identity through the loss of their stories following two centuries of colonisation. He talks about the 'power of healing in the yarn' as being about giving Aboriginal people the chance to talk about what they value, what is precious to them, as a way of healing from the trauma of loss of identity and culture. Yarning has been part of our Aboriginal and Torres Strait Islander cultures for thousands of generations. It now plays an important role, not just in research contexts, but in community contexts where telling and re-telling stories reconnects our people back to Country and culture.

## Checking-in, Checking out

At the beginning of each chapter, we ask you to 'check-in' with yourself and finish with a 'check-out' at the end of each chapter, along with some reflective questions based on the knowledge-sharing at that billabong.

The idea behind checking-in is to put your mind and your body response in focus. When we ask you to check-in, we ask you to think about how you *feel*, that is, we're asking for an *emotion*. What we're asking you to do is to stop, think, connect and be present. It doesn't matter whether or not you share this with someone else or with the group you may be in; the idea is to connect you back to yourself. For those few seconds, you're invited to activate your inquiring mind. You are also invited to connect with your body, think about what's going on for you and actually name it, which helps bring you out of that socially expected response mode. Think of the last time someone asked you how you were, and you just said "good", perhaps you weren't good at all. Think about what might have been going on for you. Did you feel safe to tell that person how you really felt? Was the person just asking without expecting a genuine response? The context and the sense of safety for the check-in becomes very important. We understand that asking people to check in with a feeling word, when they are not used to or comfortable with describing their feelings, can be quite a big thing to ask. This gets easier with practice.

For a practitioner or healer, checking-in aligns to the principle of safety in trauma therapy healing work, where we aim to support our clients to find ways to stabilise their trauma response. Regulating our own trauma response to our client's story is critical if we wish to avoid re-traumatising our clients or ourselves. This means when we work with trauma, we actively minimise our emotional responses to provide a safe space for our clients to process their trauma. You could say we are paid to *hold ourselves together*. We talk about this process more fully in Chap. 8.

**Activity 2.2 Check-in**

Take a moment to check-in with yourself now. What are you feeling? Where do you experience that feeling in your body?

**Nicole**: I'm feeling really excited to be sharing this knowledge with you. And I feel the excitement in my chest.

**Kelleigh**: I'm checking in with feeling nervous and I feel it in my stomach.

## Emotions and the Body

When we ask you to check-in and check-out, we ask you to say how you feel and where you feel that in your body. That's not always easy to do on the spot if you're not used to tuning into your body. We all have had the experience of feeling certain emotions in parts of our body and our language reflects that. When we are sad or depressed, our whole body might feel 'as heavy as lead'. When we are happy, we might feel 'light-headed'.

A group of researchers decided to investigate this emotion/body connection in more depth (Nummenmaa et al., 2014). Participants were asked to colour in two silhouettes, indicating where they felt specific emotions in response to emotional words, stories, movies or facial expressions (see Fig. 2.2). The participants were from a range of ages, cultures and backgrounds.

The researchers created body 'maps' from the hundreds of responses (see Fig. 2.3). What they found was these experiences were universal, not specific to any age or culture.

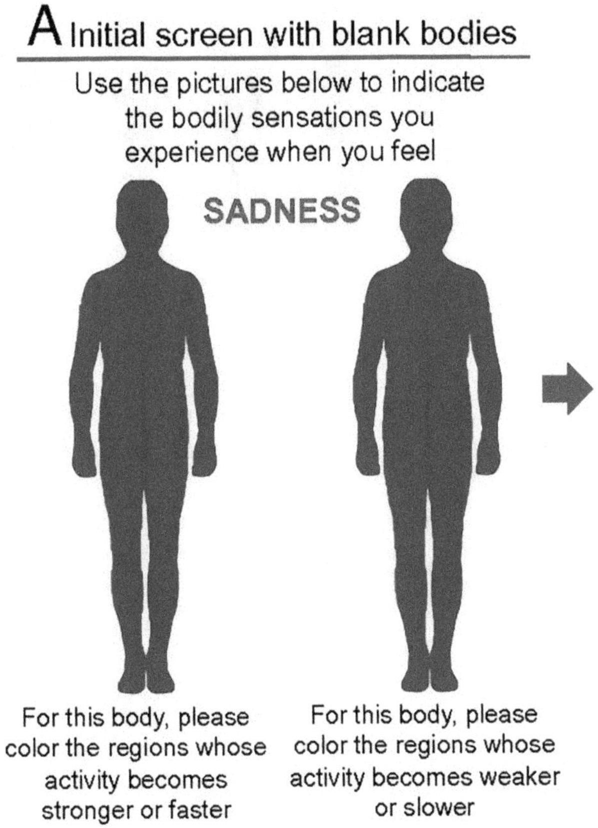


**Fig. 2.2** Emotions and the body: Initial screen with blank bodies. Source: https://www.pnas.org/content/111/2/646

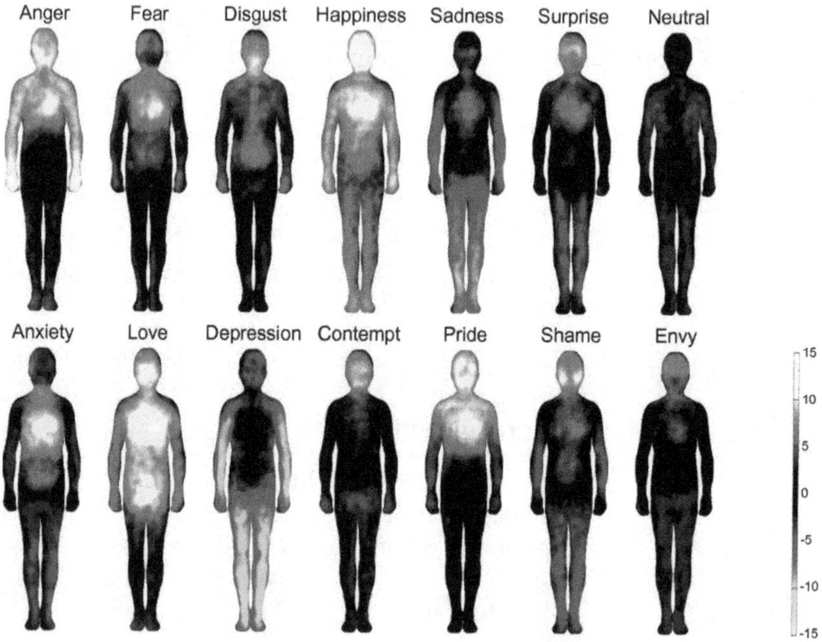


**Fig. 2.3** Maps of emotions in the body. Source: https://www.pnas.org/content/111/2/646

This short video clip from the American Museum of Natural History demonstrates in just text and sounds the main results of this research (Fig. 2.4):

In our face-to-face training we encourage our participants to use videos like these as learning tools when they work with their families and communities and clients.

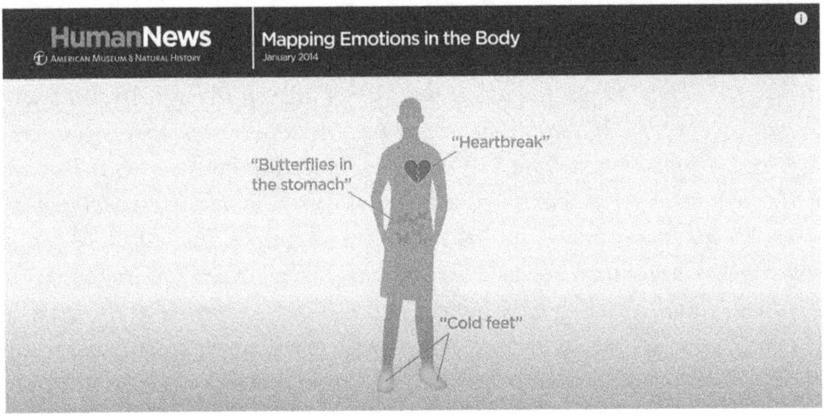


**Fig. 2.4** Mapping Emotions in the Body video. https://www.youtube.com/watch?v=cZP_I6NkQb4&feature=youtu.be&ab_channel=AmericanMuseumofNaturalHistory

### Activity 2.3 Reflective Questions on the Video

If you watched this video with someone, take some time to reflect with each other on what stood out for you. Or just write down your responses in your own time.

- What did you notice?
- What made sense?
- What surprised you?

**Kelleigh:** A few things stand out for me when I watch that clip. One is that all of those social construct feelings, like shame, embarrassment, guilt, were in the head and in the heart, whereas a lot of the deeper emotions were more embodied. They were in the body with a little bit in the head but mostly in the body, particularly depression and how cold that is all the way through.

**Nicole:** I think what really stood out for me is all the coldness in certain emotions. We often say, "I've got cold feet," when we're scared to do something. When you look at the image of someone who's feeling scared, there's no movement, no blood or anything in the feet. It's just cold. And when I think about depression, I think about how the whole body is blue and how difficult it is to come back from that place where there's nothing happening in the body.

***Kelleigh:*** *When we work with children, who often don't have language to describe how they feel, I notice what we instinctively do is say to them: "How do you feel? How do you feel about that? What are you feeling? Are you okay? What happened?" And kids don't know how to express that, they're just feeling. But if you say to a child, "Where are you feeling it? Where is it in your body? Tell me where it is that you're feeling it," they can usually say something like: "it's all in my head," or "it's all in my stomach". That can give you a much better understanding of what emotion they're actually feeling and is a good way to start peeling back some layers, looking for the rest of the story. If the child says, "it's all in my head", you might think "so the child is not really trying to communicate about anxiety. He's communicating up here. Is it fear that I'm trying to help this child with?" Given that emotional responses are quite universal, it's useful to be able to start from that understanding.*

In Chap. 4 we talk about neurological and physiological responses to threat and the systems that are activated in your body, which makes even more sense about why you feel things where you feel them. In particular, it explains why depression would be a cold feeling because often we end up in depression when we've been in hypo-arousal or exhaustion for a long time (we talk more about hyper- and hypo-arousal in Chap. 4).

This next activity gives you some experience in identifying and feeling emotions in your body.

**Activity 2.4 Feeling Emotions in the Body**

1. Let's start with *anxiety*. Imagine you're getting ready to go to a job interview, and you're starting to think about all the things you've got to remember and what you're going to say, and do you look okay, and that anxious feeling is building up inside you. Where are you feeling that anxiety in your body? Is it in your upper chest? Or your legs? Or down your spine? Just take a couple of minutes to jot down where in your body you might feel that feeling.
2. Now think about something that makes you *angry* or a recent situation where you became really angry. It might be an argument with your partner or when your kids don't clean up their rooms when you ask them. Where do you feel that anger in your body?
3. Now take a moment to imagine you're six years old. You just got ten out of ten for your first spelling test, and you just have that feeling of incredible *pride*. You did it! You're smart and you can't wait to go home and tell your family. Where do you feel that pride in your body?

## The Role of 'Grounding' Exercises

Learning about trauma can trigger a fear response to traumatic events that you, someone in your life or people you work with, may have experienced. These triggers call your body to seek safety, activating your body's nervous system into fight or flight responses. As we believe it's really important to stay safe when we share knowledge in this way, we offer examples of grounding exercises that you can take away, use on yourself, or teach to your family or your community. These can be *sensory-motor exercises*, which engage your body, *cognitive exercises,* which engage your mind, or a combination of both. These exercises help to calm your autonomic nervous system, which we talk more about in Chap. 4. These grounding exercises are very helpful any time you need to calm yourself or bring yourself back down to earth, especially if you have been triggered by trauma stories. You can also simply walk out in the sun or talk to someone as a way to self-regulate while you read through this book.

**Activity 2.5 Self-calming**

This simple exercise allows you bring yourself into the present moment and connect your mind and body. It's good to do before you head into a stressful situation or when you are feeling overwhelmed or agitated. It assists you to move from a fear response to a 'choice of presence' response, giving new context to that old fear reaction (Levine, 2010). Put your right hand on your heart and your left hand on your forehead. Close your eyes and breathe in and breathe out slowly a few times. On your out breath, release the tension in your body. Feel yourself become calm.

**Activity 2.6 Deep Breathing**

When we become hyper-aroused or anxious about something, we start breathing in a shallow way. The way to counteract that is to do some deep breathing. You may have your own ways of doing deep breathing, but this is a simple and effective method. Sometimes it's called 'divine breathing'. Breathe in for the count of six and then breathe out for the count of six. As you breathe out, crunch your tummy, which helps push the last bit of air out. Do that three or four times. If you are a First Nations person, you may wish to think of breathing in the eons of strength and connection to your ancestors and breathing out the feelings, thoughts and any heaviness in your body.

**Activity 2.7 Self-hug**

This is a good exercise to do if you're going for a job interview or going into a meeting that might be nerve-racking. If you're feeling anxious and you don't want people to see you like this, put your right hand under your left armpit (near your heart) and your left hand over your right shoulder. Give yourself a firm hug. If you do your deep breathing at the same time, it's even more powerful. The self-hug is very effective for children who are feeling anxious, because they can do it while they're going in to school or while they're waiting without anyone noticing what they're doing.

What we want to emphasise again here is that neither this book nor the training we offer is a substitute for therapy. It is knowledge sharing. Through this knowledge sharing, we hope you will support and take care of yourself. Remember that you have the power to be absolutely responsible for your own wellbeing. It's not a deficit or a weakness to take time to re-ground yourself. It's very important, not just for you, but for the work you already do or wish to do with others. Remember, we cannot draw water to nourish others if our well is dry.

## Self-Reflection as a Skill

Throughout the book, we ask you to reflect at the end of each chapter. Self-reflection is a key skill essential to the learning process. Self-reflection is about bringing your inquiring mind, your frontal cortex, your problem-solving and thinking brain back online (see Chap. 4). It's encoding all that information when you reflect on it, taking it back to your midbrain and the parts of your brain that make long-term memory. Questions like these assist the self-reflection process:

- How do you feel about that?
- What did you think about that?
- Is there something you'd like to do differently next time?
- How does this knowledge challenge your belief system?
- In what ways would this knowledge change your practice?

Being able to think about how you handled a situation, and how your worldview or knowledge system contributed to your choices, can benefit the way you work in the future. Self-reflection is therefore one of the key elements of emotional intelligence (Salovey & Mayer, 1990).

## Understanding How You Build Your Knowledge System

In this book we talk a lot about your 'knowledge system', that combination of values, beliefs and assumptions that help you make sense of the world. From the time you came into this world, you started building your knowledge system; you were told things by your parents, your teachers and your carers. Those things became your truths: you were taught what to eat; what to do; what's right; what's wrong; what will make you sick; what love and affection feel like; what's safe and what's not. From when you were in utero you were influenced by what your mother ate, her voice, the sounds of the environment you heard around you.

As you go through life, every time new knowledge presents itself, you check unconsciously and consciously on the rules of your knowledge system. As you experience the knowledge you discover at each of the billabongs, think about the effect that has on your knowledge system. You might say to yourself: "*does this fit? Yes, that makes sense". Or you may say, "no, this doesn't fit. That can't be true. That's got to be rubbish"*. And you dismiss it. We have all developed the habit of dismissing knowledge that goes against our belief systems, which are built on what we were told or exposed to as we grew up. We navigate the world according to how we *feel*, based on our rules. If something doesn't feel right, we have a conscious response to it. If the knowledge confirms our worldview, we feel good, if it doesn't, we feel threatened.

If you read something that doesn't feel right for you or makes you feel angry or makes you feel reactive in some way (and this is part of you tuning in to what's happening in your body), have a think about *why* this feels so wrong for you. What we ask of you is that when you want to dismiss something you learn about in this book, ask yourself questions like: "*Why do I find this hard to accept? Is it challenging some of the rules or beliefs that I have?* And if it's challenging those rules, ask, "*Whose knowledge system am I privileging? How did I make those rules? Whose rules was I given as a child? Do they serve me now or do I need to know more?*"

All we ask of you is to relax, open your mind, and think, "*could there be another truth that I haven't been exposed to until now? Is there another truth or new knowledge I can be open to?*" Just check in with yourself when you feel that urge to dismiss. We're not asking you to take as gospel everything we say, but we do ask you to be willing to explore more and become aware that you are feeling something and why that might be. Bring your enquiring mind to what you read, rather than just respond with a knee-jerk rejection or acceptance of the new information. These sorts of enquiring questions are the essential building blocks of critical self-reflection. The difference between an open mind and a closed mind is the level of attachment you have to the rules of your knowledge system.

Here's an example of having your knowledge system challenged that we love to use: imagine someone comes to you and says, "you know what? I've just found out that bananas are purple!" And you might say, "no way, bananas aren't purple, they're yellow!" Your knowledge system makes you sure about what's right and what's wrong; you know what colour bananas are. Then you get more information and you start hearing other people say, "well, you know, where we come from, bananas *are* purple and look, here's a picture" (Fig. 2.5). Then suddenly, your knowledge system has to change and grow to take account of this new information.

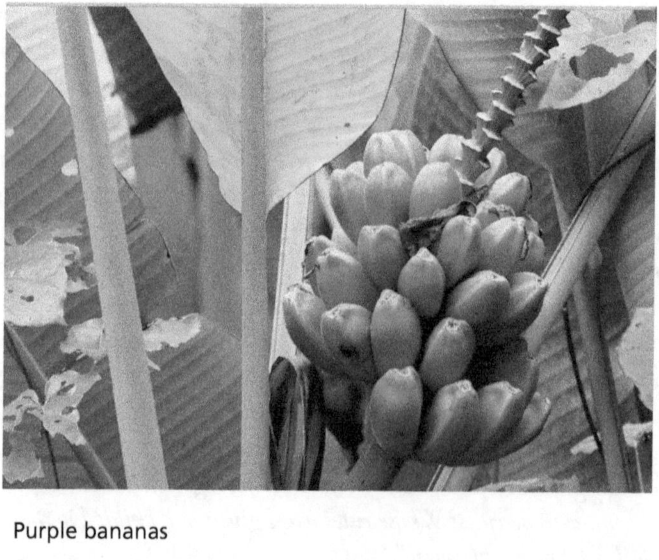

**Fig. 2.5** Purple bananas

## The Social and Emotional Wellbeing Wheel

Before we leave this billabong, we want to introduce you to a vital concept in decolonising health and well-being. When we talk about privileging Indigenous Knowledges, part of that is understanding that Aboriginal and Torres Strait Islander Peoples don't see health through the Western biomedical science model. This is at the core of trauma and healing for First Nations Peoples in Australia. A group of psychologists (Gee et al., 2014), designed a model based on Indigenous Knowledges known as the Social and Emotional Wellbeing (SEWB) Wheel (Fig. 2.6).[4] This is the holistic model that explains the way everything is connected in an Indigenous worldview.

The simplest explanation of the SEWB Wheel, is that the sections represent the essential elements of Aboriginal and Torres Strait Islander social and emotional wellbeing. For example, as connection to Country is an essential element, the lack of connection can have a significant impact on overall health. A client you're working with may present feeling unwell despite appearing to have no physical signs of illness. You may then discover that there's a big battle going on over Land Rights in their community, and realise this may be impacting on that client's overall wellbeing. We don't talk about *mental health* as such, we are more likely to talk about our *whole-self wellbeing*. Our holistic model of health existed before colonisation. This is still how Aboriginal and Torres Strait Islander Peoples think of health.

***Kelleigh***: *I often hear non-Indigenous therapists who are working with Indigenous clients say, "I'm treating this child and we're doing all these things, but it's not making a difference." And I say: "Well, what's their connection? Who's their mob? What do their families say?" And they might respond: "Well, they don't have a connection. They're not really black. They don't have that connection because they've been in care their whole life." From my point of view, I understand that all of the things that make up this human being—it doesn't matter whether they are Aboriginal or Torres Strait Islander, if their culture is missing, and what makes their wellbeing work is missing, then they can't possibly be better, because there's so many elements that aren't being fed.*

Our ancestors live in our DNA, in our Country, the air we breathe, the food that fed our people, the songlines that told us our stories of resilience and belonging. This ongoing connection was not made in one

[4]Watch the video at https://www.youtube.com/watch?v=rqLezahgmqA&ab_channel=PetrKinzel for an explanation of the wheel by one of the Aboriginal authors, Clinton Schultz.

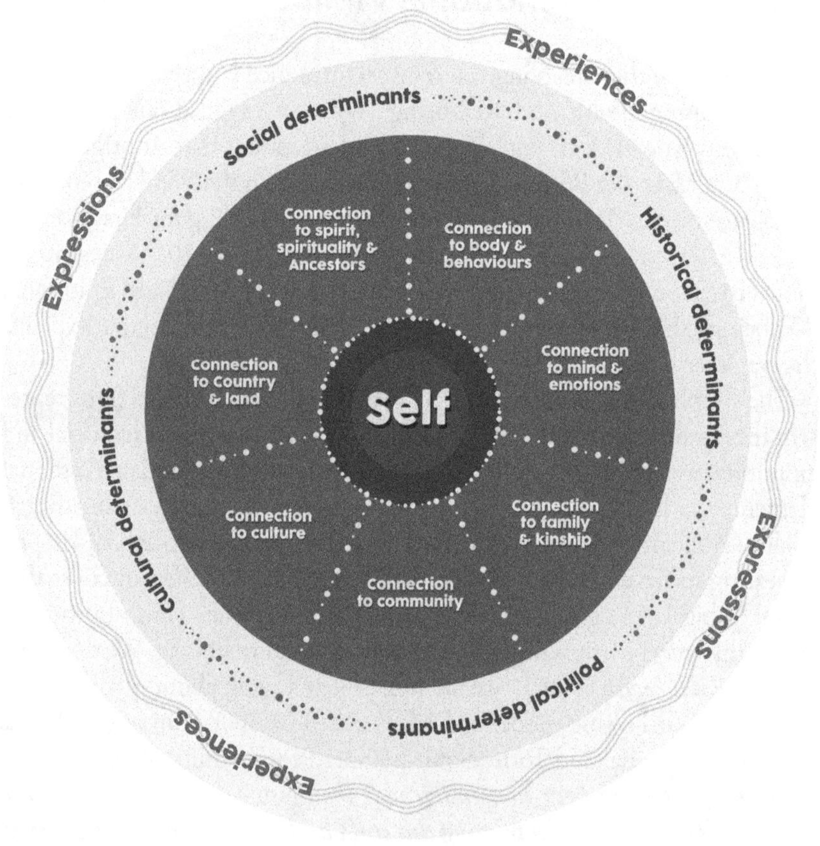


**Fig. 2.6** The social and emotional wellbeing wheel. Source: Adapted from Gee et al. (2014)

generation, but across thousands. It should not be disregarded or assumed to have disappeared because of the fracturing of the connection across a few generations as a result of colonisation.

In your DNA, in your gut, in yourself, you are likely to feel better if you eat your traditional foods, the foods of your wellbeing. In the same way, being on Country for you as an Aboriginal or Torres Strait Islander person actually makes you well (Guerin et al., 2011). We also know that *standing or walking* barefoot on the earth for a few hours per week reduces your cortisol levels, reducing your stress, which we talk more about in Chap. 4 (Kane, 2012; Roe & Aspinall, 2011; Hansen-Ketchum, 2010).

This acts more quickly than any drug. We also know that sleeping on the earth makes you feel better, even more so if you add connection to your culture and connection to your ancestors. If I'm standing, walking barefoot or lying on my Country, I am breathing the air from the trees that were nourished from my ancestors' bodies since the beginning of time.

The Social and Emotional Wellbeing Wheel is a great model to have on the wall in your office or clinic where you can start checking off all those sections and ask yourself "how is this element for my client? How is that element for this child?"

***Kelleigh***: *I find this model useful for a couple of reasons, one is when I do child protection reports. Often what I hear is "the kid doesn't have any cultural identity. They've been in care for so long and their parents were in care, so that stuff doesn't relate to them". And I say to them "just that talks so deeply to the intergenerational trauma this child has experienced." When I look at therapists' case plans, I ask them: "Where is the connection here? Tell me where and who they belong to. How long has it been since they've been home … do they know where their Country is?"*

*Also, when I work with people who are wired and stressed, I say to them: "Get yourself back to Country, wherever that is. If you're a saltwater person, find your way to the saltwater. It's really important." The elements of the SEWB Wheel are the things I now ask for clinicians to consider having in their reports. This is how we look at health. I say: "if they're not in your case plan, if they're not in your report, if they're not in the way you talk with your client, then you're missing something, and you are doing yourself and your client a disservice".*

Connection to country can look like many different things for different people. For example, while you might be treating the child, what's going on in their family group, in their clan, in their community, is really important for their wellbeing. This is similar to the Western 'nested systems theory' (Neal & Neal, 2013). If we've got children whose parents or whose families have been moved off Country, or where there's a dam on their Country where they once would have practised ceremony, how do they practice cultural activities now? If you are a First Nations person living in the city, consider when the last time was that you listened to the drums or clapsticks, used language or sat and listened to an Elder. Consider also that there are many different levels of understanding and identifying as an Aboriginal or Torres Strait Islander person. Where the person is on that journey will determine what cultural connections they may seek out. For some, connection to country might be as simple as finding out who your mob are and where they are from.

**Activity 2.8 Your Strengths**

- What do you see as your main strengths?
- What are the most significant contributors to your sense of cultural, social and emotional wellbeing?
- Who may have passed these strengths on to you?

## Concluding Comments

We have begun the journey into cultural safety in trauma-informed practice. At the next billabong, we unpack the ideas and concepts related to what it means to be culturally safe in First Nations contexts and practice. Take time to check-out and reflect on what you have taken from this billabong.

**Activity 2.9 Check-out and Reflection**

Consider these questions:

- How are you feeling now in your body?
- What stories spoke to your heart?
- What challenged your belief system?
- What will you do now to take care of yourself?
- How could you use the knowledge you've taken from this billabong in your life and work?

## References and Further Reading

Barlo, S. (2016). *Can the impacts of colonisation on the dignity of Aboriginal men be reversed?* (PhD), Southern Cross University, Lismore.

Barlo, S., Boyd, W. E., Pelizzon, A., & Wilson, S. (2020). Yarning as protected space: Principles and protocols. *AlterNative: An International Journal of Indigenous Peoples, 16*(2), 90–98.

Belfrage, M. (2007). Why "culturally safe" health care? *Medical Journal of Australia, 186*(10), 537–538. https://doi.org/10.5694/j.1326-5377.2007.tb01032.x

Bessarab, D., & Ng'andu, B. (2010). Yarning about yarning as a legitimate method in Indigenous research. *International Journal of Critical Indigenous Studies, 3*(1), 37–50.

Fredericks, B., Adams, K., Finlay, S., Fletcher, G., Andy, S., Briggs, L., Hall, R., et al. (2011). Engaging the practice of Indigenous yarning in action research. *ALAR: Action Learning and Action Research Journal, 17*(2), 12–24.

Gee, G., Dudgeon, P., Schultz, C., Hart, A., & Kelly, K. (2014). Aboriginal and Torres Strait Islander social and emotional wellbeing. In P. Dudgeon, H. Milroy, & R. Walker (Eds.), *Working together: Aboriginal and Torres Strait Islander mental health and wellbeing principles and practice* (pp. 55–68). Commonwealth of Australia.

Geia, L. K., Hayes, B., & Usher, K. (2013). Yarning/Aboriginal storytelling: Towards an understanding of an Indigenous perspective and its implications for research practice. *Contemporary Nurse, 46*(1), 13–17. https://doi.org/10.5172/conu.2013.46.1.13

Guerin, P., Guerin, B., Tedmanson, D., & Clark, Y. (2011). How can country, spirituality, music and arts contribute to Indigenous mental health and well-being? *Australasian Psychiatry, 19*(Suppl 1), S38–S41. https://doi.org/10.3109/10398562.2011.583065

Hansen-Ketchum, P. A. (2010). *Engaging with Nature: A Participatory Study in the Promotion of Health.* (PhD), University of Alberta.

Howlett, J. R., & Paulus, M. P. (2015). The neural basis of testable and non-testable beliefs. *PLoS One, 10*(5), e0124596–e0124596. https://doi.org/10.1371/journal.pone.0124596

Hughes, M., & Barlo, S. (2020). Yarning with country: An indigenist research methodology. *Qualitative Inquiry, 27*(3–4), 353–363. https://doi.org/10.1177/1077800420918889

Jacks, J. Z., & Cameron, K. A. (2003). Strategies for resisting persuasion. *Basic and Applied Social Psychology, 25*(2), 145–161. https://doi.org/10.1207/S15324834BASP2502_5

Kane, E. (2012). Feet on the ground. *Better Nutrition, 74*(12), 22–23.

Jackson-Barrett, E., Price, A., Stomski, N., & Walker, B. F. (2015). Grounded in country: Perspectives on working within, alongside and for Aboriginal communities. *Issues in Educational Research, 25*(1), 36–49. Retrieved from https://ezproxy.scu.edu.au/login?url=https://search.ebscohost.com/login.aspx?direct=true&db=ehh&AN=102382766&site=ehost-live

Lawrence, R. L., & Paige, D. S. (2016). What our ancestors knew: Teaching and learning through storytelling. *New Directions for Adult and Continuing Education, 149*(6), 63–72.

Levine, P. A. (2010). *In an unspoken voice: How the body releases trauma and restores goodness.* North Atlantic Books.

Lin, I., Green, C., & Bessarab, D. (2016). 'Yarn with me': Applying clinical yarning to improve clinician–patient communication in Aboriginal health care. *Australian Journal of Primary Health, 22*(5), 377–382. https://doi.org/10.1071/PY16051

Martin, K. L. (2008). *Please knock before you enter: Aboriginal regulation of outsiders and the implications for researchers*. Post Pressed.

Neal, J. W., & Neal, Z. P. (2013). Nested or networked? Future directions for ecological systems theory. *Social Development, 22*(4), 722–737.

Neale, M., & Kelly, L. (2020). *Songlines: The power and promise*. Thames & Hudson.

Nummenmaa, L., Glerean, E., Hari, R., & Hietanen, J. K. (2014). Bodily maps of emotions. *Proceedings of the National Academy of Sciences, 111*(2), 646–651. https://doi.org/10.1073/pnas.1321664111

Rigney, L.-I. (1999). Internationalization of an Indigenous anticolonial cultural critique of research methodologies: A guide to Indigenist research methodology and its principles. *Wicazo Sa Review, 14*(2), 109–121.

Roe, J., & Aspinall, P. (2011). The restorative benefits of walking in urban and rural settings in adults with good and poor mental health. *Health & Place, 17*(1), 103–113.

Salovey, P., & Mayer, J. D. (1990). Emotional intelligence. *Imagination, Cognition and Personality, 9*(3), 185–211.

Salzman, M. B. (2018). Cultural trauma and recovery. In M. B. Salzman (Ed.), *A psychology of culture* (pp. 67–78). Springer International Publishing.

Smith, L. T. (1999). *Decolonizing methodologies: Research and indigenous peoples*. St Martin's.

Somerville, C., Somerville, K., & Wyld, F. (2010). Martu storytellers: Aboriginal narratives within the academy. *The Australian Journal of Indigenous Education, 39*(S1), 96–102.

Terare, M., & Rawsthorne, M. (2020). Country is yarning to me: Worldview, health and well-being amongst Australian First Nations People. *The British Journal of Social Work, 50*(3), 944–960. https://doi.org/10.1093/bjsw/bcz072

Towney, L. M. (2005). The power of healing in the yarn: Working with Aboriginal men. *International Journal of Narrative Therapy & Community Work, 2005*(1), 39–43.

Walker, M., Fredericks, B., Mills, K., & Anderson, D. (2014). "Yarning" as a method for community-based health research with Indigenous women: The indigenous women's wellness research program. *Health Care for Women International, 35*(10), 1216–1226.

Whitfield-Gabrieli, S., Moran, J. M., Nieto-Castañón, A., Triantafyllou, C., Saxe, R., & Gabrieli, J. D. E. (2011). Associations and dissociations between default and self-reference networks in the human brain. *NeuroImage, 55*(1), 225–232. https://doi.org/10.1016/j.neuroimage.2010.11.048

Yunkaporta, T., & Kirby, M. (2011). Yarning up Aboriginal pedagogies: A dialogue about eight Aboriginal ways of learning. In N. Purdie, G. Milgate, & H. R. Bell (Eds.), *Two way teaching and learning: Toward culturally reflective and relevant education* (pp. 205–213). ACER Press.

Yunkaporta, T., & McGinty, S. (2009). Reclaiming Aboriginal knowledge at the cultural interface. *Australian Educational Researcher, 36*(2), 55–72.

# 3

# Towards Cultural Safety: Cultural Safety in Trauma-Informed Practice from an Indigenous Perspective

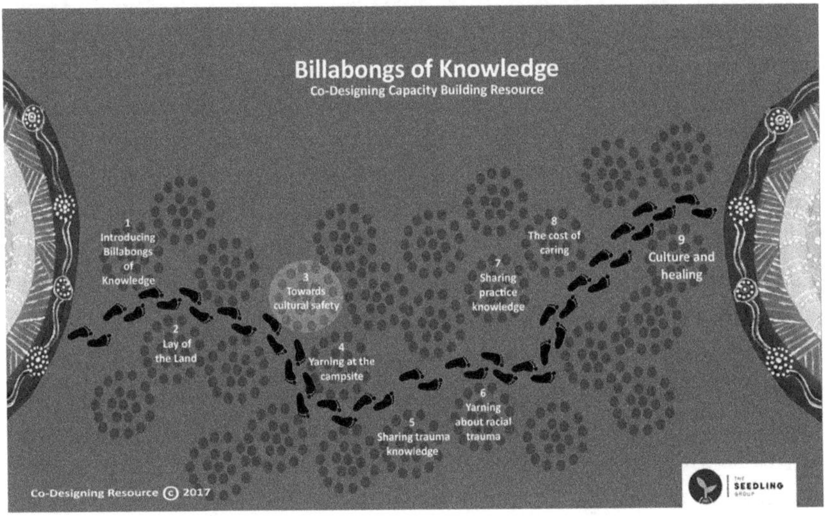


I would like to acknowledge and pay my deepest respects to the Country that I am privileged to work and live on, as well as Elders and community who are of this country. I also pay my deepest respects and gratitude to my traditional Country, Elders and community. I thank all of our Ancestors collectively for the privilege of bringing us here to this place and time today.

Stacey Vervoort, Gamilaroi psychologist



N. Tujague, K. Ryan, *Cultural Safety in Trauma-Informed Practice from a First Nations Perspective*, https://doi.org/10.1007/978-3-031-13138-7_3

This book is about *cultural safety* in trauma-informed practice and is written from an Indigenous perspective. At this billabong we define what cultural safety is, looking through a trauma-informed lens. We talk about our understanding of a *holistic* concept of the individual on a cellular, spiritual, psychological, emotional, cultural, environmental and political level. Our aim is to make visible the complexities of all these connected and interdependent levels when we think about health and healing. The first step in any trauma-informed practice is to ensure *safety*. How can we understand how to provide 'safety' if we do not know what values and meanings underpin a client's cultural view of what safety means to them? It is most likely not possible to achieve complete culturally safe practice in colonised contexts; we can only move towards it.

It is only when ideas of cultural safety combine First Nations and non-Indigenous healing knowledges, that we can begin to repair the complex injury that comes from collective trauma. We pay our respects to the many healing modalities, ceremonies and practices used by First Nations cultures around the world. We avoid the use of any one discipline-specific language, preferring to explain concepts and terms that have universal meaning and are authentic in our meaning making as First Nations Australians. At this billabong we yarn about the variety of terms used as part of the cultural safety continuum, including 'cultural awareness', 'cultural competence ', 'cultural sensitivity', 'cultural appropriateness,' 'cultural responsiveness', 'cultural humility', 'cultural security', 'cultural respect, 'cultural courage', and 'cultural intelligence'. All these different terms can be a bit confusing for everybody, including Aboriginal and Torres Strait Islander Peoples. We discuss how important it is to view cultural safety through a trauma lens as well as learning more about your own culture and your cultural worldview.

First, let's start with a check-in …

### Activity 3.1 Check in

We often use these Bear Cards (Fig. 3.1) in our face-to-face training for check-ins because we find it's an effective way of connecting with and naming how you feel right now. Most of us aren't very good at recognising what we are experiencing in our body, probably because we spend so much time in our heads.

Nicole: I'll choose a calm bear today with his hands on his tummy because I'm calm and looking forward to yarning about a few important ideas.

Kelleigh: I would choose that bear with his hands crossed because I'm feeling curious: where will this conversation take us today?

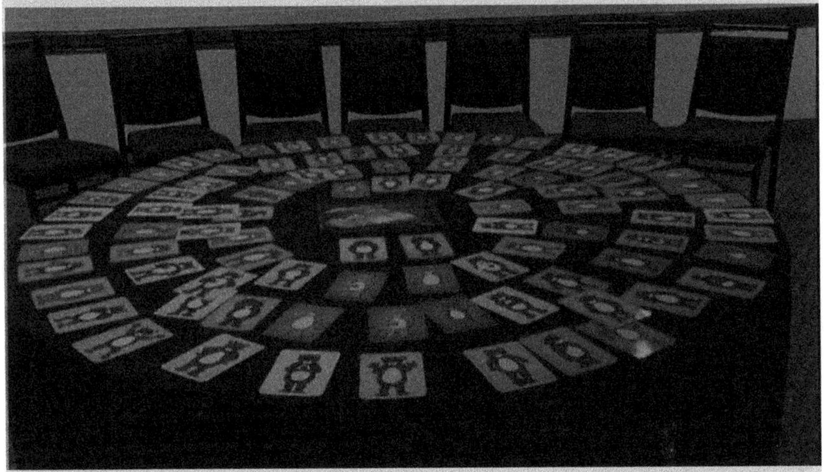

**Fig. 3.1** Bear cards (Check out this website for digital versions of the cards: https://innovativeresources.org/resources/digital-applications/bears-digital-version/). Source: photo taken at one of our trainings

**Activity 3.2 Breathing Exercise**

Take a moment to tune in to how you're feeling in your mind and in your body today. Have you been rushing around before you settled down to read? Have you been in meetings all morning or had a late night? Just take some time now to focus on what's going on in your body and how you're feeling. If you're feeling like you're a bit hunched up and you've been rushing, take some nice deep breaths, bring your shoulders down away from your ears and get yourself into a nice, relaxed position and allow your mind to calm. Take a long deep breath in through your nose while counting to 4 and breathe out through your mouth for the count of 6, crunching your tummy muscles to release the last bit of air and tension from your lungs. Breathe in through your nose again for the count of 4 and out through your mouth for the count of 6. Do this a few times until you feel yourself calming and relaxing. (What you have just done can be recognised as a *sensory-motor* exercise).

Before we go any further, we would like to remind you about the importance of keeping mind and body together in harmony (see Chap. 8 for more information about the importance of self-care). Checking in aims to restore balance to body, mind and spirit to keep you safe while you share this knowledge.

## An Indigenous Perspective on Cultural Safety

Many Indigenous Peoples think of collective social and emotional wellbeing as including connection to past, present and future. If you are a practitioner, it is important to collaborate across multiple worldviews to be effective and make a difference in an Indigenous health and wellbeing context. Providing culturally safe practice and using a trauma-informed lens opens another whole layer of understanding for both you and your clients. It is important to appreciate what is valued and important for the *whole self* of each person. For Aboriginal and Torres Strait Islander Peoples in Australia, this means hearing a person's *whole* story, even if it goes back many generations. Looking through a trauma lens means changing your focus from a deficit model of what's *wrong* with that person to a strengths-based model of *what is the story* of that person.

This holistic or *whole of story* understanding comes through combining Indigenous and non-Indigenous healing knowledges to build a treatment plan that is culturally safe. Incorporating the trauma knowledge of each worldview supports healing for both the individual *and* the community. Nature and science have shown us that any untended wound leaves unresolved injury which can manifest in other ways. These untended wounds allow unresolved pain, loss and grief to continue for the individual and the community. It is only through decolonising the assumed privilege of the non-Indigenous model of health and healing that we can provide genuine culturally safe healing (Reyes Cruz & Sonn, 2011).

***Kelleigh***: *I like to tell the story of the magpie when I talk about respecting different worldviews. The magpie does not compare her song with that of the crow, for the voice of the magpie is meant for her family, and the voice of the crow is meant for her family. Each is respectful of and respected by all creatures. But the message of the magpie is meant for those whose way is that of the magpie...*

When you think about this story, reflect on what we talked about in Chap. 2 about worldviews. Whose voice is privileged? It is the magpie's worldview, language, knowledge system, *her* ways of being and doing. If you are not of the magpie, you need to learn stuff; if you don't understand her way you run the risk of making mistakes. It doesn't mean that the *magpie* needs to change so she can talk to you. *You* need to understand there's a whole other worldview going on here.

## Defining Cultural Safety: A Continuum of Practices

The term 'cultural safety' was first used when Māori nurse and scholar Irihapeti Ramsden (Papps & Ramsden, 1996; Ramsden, 2002) suggested that non-Indigenous New Zealand nurses needed to develop skills to be able to deal with patients from different cultures in a more culturally safe way. Ramsden's work grew out of her observation that only one worldview was being used to train nurses and only one knowledge system influenced that training. It was not the knowledge system of the patients who were the receiving the treatment. When the Nursing Council of New Zealand made cultural safety a compulsory component of nursing and midwifery courses in 1992, which was a direct result of Ramsden's work (Papps & Ramsden, 1996), it began a new way of looking at individuals and their cultural needs. Cultural safety up until that point had been verging on stereotyping of cultures and their beliefs rather than recognising the many facets of different cultures.

The definition of 'cultural safety' used by the Nursing Council at the time was:

> The effective nursing of a person/family of another culture by a nurse who has undertaken a process of personal reflection on own cultural identity and recognises the impact of the nurses' culture on own nursing practice (Papps & Ramsden, 1996, p. 491).

The strongest current definition we have come across is that articulated in a report by the Australian Evaluation Society. It privileges the experience of First Nations Peoples over that of non-Indigenous practitioners and describes what an ideal culturally safe situation would look like from a First Nations point of view:

> Cultural safety is an experience determined by First Nations peoples when they are in situations where their presence is welcomed and respected, their experiences are believed and validated, their cultures are centred and valued, their knowledges and skills are recognised and supported, their advice is listened to and acted upon, and they do not experience racism in any form (Gollan & Stacey, 2021, p. 39).

The whole idea of 'cultural safety' in a mainstream health context has grown from a practice used by nurses in Aotearoa to becoming almost a discipline in itself, spreading out across the world to other professions such as psychology, medicine, social work, education and law, each with their own preferred terms and practices. We can think of these terms as placed on a continuum, progressing from cultural awareness, through cultural competence and finally to cultural safety, which ideally encompasses all the features of the range of terms we discuss briefly in the 'Want to know more…?' section below. Irihapeti Ramsden was the first to conceptualise this continuum when she initiated discussions about cultural safety in nursing in New Zealand (Ramsden, 1992, 2002).

## Want to know more about terms on the cultural safety continuum?

Since Irihapeti Ramsden (1992) first introduced the term 'cultural safety', there has been a proliferation of related terms that 'reflects not only the multidimensional and dynamic nature of culture but also the countless ways in which culture has been conceptualized' (Danso, 2018, p. 412). Here we take a closer look at the more common terms used in cross-cultural (also called 'transcultural' or 'intercultural') contexts, particularly as they relate to First Nations peoples who have experienced the trauma of colonisation. These include terms such as: cultural awareness, cultural competence, cultural sensitivity, cultural security, cultural respect, cultural appropriateness, cultural responsiveness, cultural humility, cultural courage and cultural intelligence.

Most of the literature dealing with terms on the cultural safety continuum comes from the fields of healthcare (especially nursing and midwifery), medicine, allied health, social work, counselling, education and psychology. A useful resource is Danso (2018), who summarises the main features of some of the terms we cover in this section, namely cultural awareness, cultural sensitivity, cultural appropriateness, cultural safety, cultural competence and cultural humility.

**Cultural awareness**

Training in 'cultural awareness' is very common and considered a minimum requirement for people who work in culturally diverse contexts. The main focus of these programs is to increase awareness of the cultural, social and historical factors behind Indigenous peoples' experience and to encourage participants to be self-reflective about their own culture, possible biases and tendency to stereotype (Thomson, 2005). The assumptions behind this training are to help workers become more 'tolerant' and then adjust their practice accordingly when they work with First Nations people (Downing et al., 2011). The limitations of this approach are well-expressed by Aboriginal scholar Bronwyn Fredericks:

> The mere creation of awareness does not bring about the structural changes needed and the recognition of our inherent Indigenous rights, nor the reflection on the positioning of Indigenous people by non-Indigenous people. It does not mean that participants will look at their own subjective identity in relationship to the social order. ... It does not mean that we as Indigenous peoples will be any healthier, as defined by Indigenous people. It does not mean that we will be exercising our rights, roles and responsibilities as Indigenous peoples or that non-Indigenous people will be exploring how they acquired their privileged positioning within Australia and move to re-dress their positioning (Fredericks, 2008, p. 87).

(*continued*)

**(continued)**

**Cultural competence**

In the literature, you'll find a range of definitions of the concept of cultural competence. Cultural competence training (also called 'diversity training', 'cross-cultural training' or 'multicultural training') aims to improve health workers' awareness, knowledge and skills so that they can 'manage' cultural factors in relation to health service interventions (Downing et al., 2011). It requires people who work with people from cultures other than the mainstream culture to develop awareness of their own cultural values, beliefs, and biases; develop knowledge of the values and beliefs of the cultural group they are working with; acknowledge cultural diversity as a resource and not as a 'problem' to overcome; and acknowledge culture as being' fluid and dynamic' (Danso, 2018 p. 413).

Cultural competence training has been criticised for not going far enough in holding workers accountable for the privilege and power of their position, which contributes to the failure to address the unequal power relations between Aboriginal and non-Aboriginal people. Critics also claim that such training tends to be tokenistic and there is little evidence that Indigenous cultural competence training changes practice (Herring et al., 2013; Curtis et al., 2019). Two significant limitations that are relevant for our work are that cultural competence training 'does not address the ongoing trauma legacies from invasion, and ... does not take account of the ongoing experiences of racism experienced by Aboriginal people' (Herring et al., 2013, p. 107).

**Cultural sensitivity**

American nursing scholar Jacqueline Burchum (2002) sees cultural sensitivity as one of the attributes of cultural competence. The 'dimensions' of this attribute include appreciating and valuing diversity, appreciating and respecting each client's beliefs and values, genuinely caring about people from other cultures and appreciating 'how one's own cultural background may influence professional practice' (p. 8). Canadian nursing scholars Annette Browne and Colleen Varcoe (2006) look at the limitations of these notions of cultural sensitivity in relation to health care involving (Canadian) Aboriginal peoples. They argue that the kinds of 'cultural traits' (values, beliefs and practices) identified in the types of definition above, 'are typically those that are identified as different from "ours" with the unspoken comparison being with the assumed dominant norm' (Browne & Varcoe, 2006, p. 158). They go on to suggest that currently, 'both within the wider society and in health care more specifically, culture continues to be used as synonymous with difference—differences that are most often based on stereotypes' (p. 159). Furthermore, they argue that these understandings of cultural sensitivity are founded on liberal ideas of 'tolerance', which means that seemingly well-meaning expressions of 'respect and even appreciation of Aboriginal peoples' culture can sometimes mask the racialized assumptions embedded in such discourses' (p. 160).

(*continued*)

**(continued)**

**Cultural security**

The 'cultural security' model was developed in Australia as a response to the limitations of cultural awareness and cultural competence training. It emphasises that the responsibility for providing culturally secure health services lies with the system as a whole, not the individual health worker (Downing et al., 2011, pp. 249–250). It is also about incorporating cultural values into the design, delivery and evaluation of services. It is designed to 'effect change in all elements of the health system: workforce development, workforce reform, purchasing of health services, monitoring and accountability, and public engagement' (Farrelly & Lumby, 2009, p. 14).

**Cultural respect**

The broad term of 'cultural respect' was defined by the Australian Health Ministers Advisory Council in 2004 as "Recognition, protection and continued advancement of the inherent rights, cultures and traditions of Aboriginal and Torres Strait Islander peoples", noting that cultural respect can only be achieved when health service providers create an environment in which cultural differences are respected, and Indigenous peoples can feel culturally safe (cited in Farrelly & Lumby, 2009, p. 15). As with 'cultural security', none of the available cultural respect literature provides direction on how cultural training will achieve this goal (Downing et al., 2011)

**Cultural appropriateness**

Interventions or programs are considered 'culturally appropriate' if they ensure services reflect local traditions and suit the cultural context; acknowledge historical experiences of colonisation and oppression; and recognise First Nations peoples' unique characteristics and needs (Danso, 2018 p. 413). One study (Smith et al., 2017) aimed to compare the perceptions of Australian Aboriginal community members and primary health care (PHC) providers in remote North West Queensland about the cultural appropriateness of the provision and delivery of health services. One significant finding was that while 85% of the PHC providers 'perceived that communication between them and Aboriginal patients was clear and understandable, only half of the Aboriginal community members (46.3%) agreed with that' (Smith et al., 2017, pp. 237–238).

**Cultural responsiveness**

Cultural responsiveness is a term used primarily in pedagogical frameworks, such as in the disciplines of social work education (Bennett & Gates, 2019; Bennett et al., 2018; Harris & O'Donoghue, 2020), teacher education (Daniels-Mayes, 2019); and allied health education programs such as physiotherapy (Te et al., 2019). According to Bennett & Gates, cultural responsiveness is 'an ongoing process that requires awareness of the relationship between ourselves and others and the systems in which we interact' (2019, p. 606). Given the colonised context in which Australian social work education and practice are situated, Bennett et al. (2018) argue that:

*(continued)*

**(continued)**

> if social work students are to make room for new ways of knowing, being and doing in their practice, they need to make critical ontological, epistemological and political shifts in their understandings of themselves and their practice contexts. This requires embracing the power of not knowing, of sitting with uncertainty and being willing to be challenged and shaped by these 'different' ways of knowing (p. 813).

Similarly, in the teacher education context, Daniels-Mayes, an Australian Aboriginal teacher-educator, argues that 'to be a successful, confident, culturally responsive teacher with Aboriginal students, pre-service teachers need to courageously interrogate their own, and society's, embedded racialised narratives' (Daniels-Mayes, 2019, p. 540). She uses a method of 'counterstorytelling' with her students which is 'both a method of telling stories of experiences that are not often told as well as a tool for critiquing the stories of those in power and whose story is a normalised part of the dominant narrative' (p. 541). We encourage you to follow up this paper to see how this talented educator conducts a creative conversation with 'Master Racism' as a character.

**Cultural humility**

Cultural humility was a term first used in the medical context as a tool for training physicians in the delivery of culturally appropriate medical care (Danso, 2018). It was defined then as:

> a lifelong commitment to self-evaluation and critique, to redressing the power imbalances in the physician-patient dynamic, and to developing mutually beneficial and non-paternalistic partnerships with communities on behalf of individuals and defined populations (Tervalon & Murray-Garcia, 1998, p. 123).

However, this concept has mainly been applied in the field of social work (Bennett & Gates, 2019; Campinha-Bacote, 2019; Danso, 2018; Fisher-Borne et al., 2015; Foronda et al., 2016; Harris & O'Donoghue, 2020; Ortega & Faller, 2011; Rosen et al., 2017). A fundamental assumption of cultural humility is that being culturally humble automatically translates into respect for diversity, where 'deliberate acts of self-analysis move... beyond tolerating difference to developing a capacity for minority empowerment' (Danso, 2018, p. 424). The following definition summarises its main elements:

*(continued)*

**(continued)**

> The cultural humility approach includes three core elements: institutional and individual accountability; lifelong learning and critical reflection; and mitigating power imbalances... at the core of cultural humility is a sense of accountability, which differs immensely from a sense of mastery. Accountability means a commitment to self-reflection that is active and responsible (Fisher-Borne et al., 2015, p. 174).

Critics such as Danso (2018) argue that while cultural humility 'sounds linguistically appealing [it] lacks conceptual clarity and definitional unanimity among its advocates and even the term humility is not clearly defined' (p. 424)

**Cultural courage**

Closely aligned with cultural humility is the concept of 'cultural courage', again mainly used by social workers. Having cultural courage 'enables social workers to interact with and be guided by Aboriginal knowledge and worldviews rather than imposing their own prejudices on the situation' (Fernando & Bennett, 2018, p. 55). For non-Aboriginal social workers, it means:

> having an ability to understand how their own cultural background, privilege, values, and assumptions impact on how they relate to people. It also encompasses the need to acknowledge and confront fears, uncertainties, and anxieties that can arise in practice and to resist the temptation of becoming immobilised. For Indigenous workers, developing cultural courage involves the need to reflect on their own experiences of racism and history of colonisation and how this impacts on their work (Bennett et al., 2011, p. 34).

**Cultural intelligence**

'Cultural intelligence' (Edwards, 2016) is worthwhile mentioning here as a term used in social work circles in the US. Edwards, a female African American scholar, draws on her own experience of 'racial microaggressions' (see Chap. 5) in the academy, suggesting this concept could be valuable in the development of social worker identity in cross-cultural interactions. Briefly, this cross-cultural competency requires knowledge of cross-cultural phenomena (process knowledge), reflective mindfulness (key to connecting knowledge with action) and behavioural skills that demonstrate flexibility in cross-cultural interactions. Edwards refers to the work of African American author W.E.B. Du Bois, who wrote in his treatise The Souls of Black Folk (1903) about his people needing to have a 'double consciousness'. African Americans need to 'see themselves from the perspective of both cultures [resulting in]...having more than one social identity' (Edwards, 2016, p. 218). This is similar to what Aboriginal and Torres Strait Islander Peoples call 'walking in both worlds'.

## Cultural Safety Requires a Trauma Lens

Throughout this book, we investigate why it's very difficult to work in a culturally safe way if you don't understand the impacts of trauma on the brain and body. What struck us when we investigated all the terms we talk about in the previous section is the obvious absence in the literature of the link between cultural safety and the understanding of trauma. We put the case in a recent paper (Tujague & Ryan, 2021) that it's just not possible to be culturally safe if you don't have a trauma lens. Indigenous-led cultural safety training is an essential foundation to give us guidelines and knowledge. This is best delivered by Traditional Owners of the nation where you are doing your work. Adhering to cultural checklists may be a good beginning to understanding cultural safety, however, to heal the long-term effects of historical trauma your practice needs to be underpinned by a trauma-informed lens (see Chap. 5).

If you have learned about the history of the people you're working with and if you look through a trauma lens, you may see the behaviours of your clients in a different light. Psychologists and sociologists may call some of those behaviours 'deviant', meaning different from the 'norm' or what is expected by mainstream society. The deficit approach pathologises those behaviours.

When you recognise that the behaviours you're seeing are strategies that people have learned in order to survive in the environment they're living in, or ways to cope and live given the trauma they've experienced, then you'll understand that it's not *deviant* behaviour, it's *trauma or threat response* behaviour. What you have there is an activated nervous system that's acting out, trying to keep safe. (We talk more about how trauma responses are activated in Chap. 4).

## Know Your Own Cultural Worldview

If we go back to that original definition of cultural safety in the New Zealand nursing context, the emphasis is on the nurse's "personal reflection on own cultural identity". You cannot be culturally safe unless you know your own culture, unless you know what it is about your culture that's different from the culture of the person or people you're working with. The worldview you bring to the situation influences what information you will attend to and what you dismiss. The treatment plan you'll formulate and what support networks you'll activate, will only be appropriate if you know what's been going on, not only for the individual, but for the family and community.

***Kelleigh:*** *If I am a saltwater person, I might say that culture is like the saltwater air I breathe, the skip of my heart at the beat of the island drums or the sound of the waves on the shore. It might be the familiar sounds of language, the respect I feel, my desire to be part of the clan gathering. It is in my DNA and in my consciousness, all-knowing, but unsaid. It includes ceremony, rituals, practices and belonging. A friend from the Torres Strait once told me, "Culture and me, we are like the fish and the water".*

You may be a non-Indigenous person who thinks, "well, I don't actually have a culture." But you *do* have your own culture, which can take a little bit of unpacking when you are part of the dominant or mainstream culture. The reflective questions at the end of this chapter may be helpful in this process of unpacking.

***Nicole****: I would like to tell you a story about how I really was challenged by my own cultural worldview. Our great grandfather was one of those taken from Gaua Island in Vanuatu, to come and work the cane fields in North Queensland. When we as a family went back to Vanuatu to connect with this side of our family, we flew to a small island where we caught a boat to a village around the other side of the bay. It was a long trip. We slept in bamboo huts that were built especially for us. It was an amazing experience for us all.*

*At the end of our visit, we went down to the water's edge while we were waiting for the boat to come and pick us up. We watched the local kids playing in the water. They were spearing things, picking up things, building fires, cooking things. I couldn't quite see as I didn't have my glasses on and I said to my sisters, "what are the kids playing with down there?" Our little sister Riley walked down to where they were playing and came back and she said, "OK, don't go down to the water's edge." Of course, as soon as anyone says something like that, you've just got to go and have a look.*

*What the kids were playing with were these little pre-born piglets. I was shocked and walked back and said to our brother Chris, "the kids are playing with little pre-born piglets!" (Fig. 3.2) He said, "well, we've got Toys R Us and these kids*

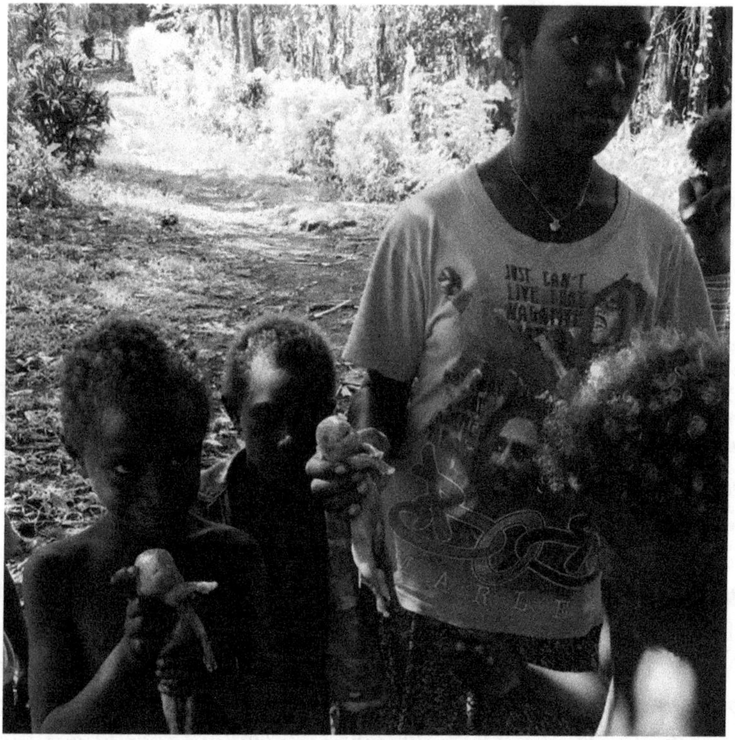

**Fig. 3.2** Pre-born piglets, Gaua Island, Vanuatu. Source: Photo taken by Nicole Tujague, used with permission from the families

*have piglets." I thought "our family here don't use toys and books like we do at home in Australia, so how do they learn about what baby piglets look like? How do they learn about fishing and spearing and cooking things? This is how they learn."*

*That was such an important lesson for me about my cultural worldview, how I was comparing the Gaua Island culture (which is my cultural heritage too) to my mainstream cultural perspective. The lesson in that story is that we all have different cultures that we bring to the table and being aware of that helps us develop cultural awareness and become more culturally safe. Kelleigh has another perspective on this story that gives more context.*

***Kelleigh:*** *The backstory to what we saw the kids doing at the water's edge is that there had been a death and a burial ceremony or funeral, what*

*Aboriginal and Torres Strait Islander Peoples call 'sorry business'. The people in the community were preparing for the funeral feast. The older boy was being taught how to kill the animal and how to prepare it for the feast. Unfortunately, in his exuberance about being given the honour of this responsibility, he killed the wrong animal. He killed a female pig and she was pregnant with piglets. This was not a small mistake, as a pregnant female pig is a very big asset to a small community.*

*But instead of the boy getting in trouble and being punished, the adults explained to him what had happened and how he had made the mistake. They saw no benefit in punishing him, but instead took the opportunity to teach him. Then they made use of everything: the pig was eaten; the piglets were used to teach the kids about birth, about growing, about the connection with everything. There was no deficit model operating here at all. It was all about learning, and learning from everything that happened, especially mistakes, unlike in our school system's deficit model, where you either get it or you don't, where if you do something wrong you are punished for that mistake. On the Island that day, because the boy did something that was unexpected, everyone could learn from it. But when you are punished, you only respond to threat, and you can't learn when you are in that threat response.*

*The lesson for me that struck a chord that day was about different cultures and how we teach, which is so important when we are talking about cultural worldviews: there is no such thing as reality, there is only perception. If you think that what you know is all about 'reality', you are only talking about the meaning from the perspective of your own worldview.*

## Concluding Comments

At the next couple of billabongs, we'll take a closer look at the brain and the nervous system, how they respond when we're experiencing trauma or we're working with someone who's experiencing trauma. We finish off our stay at this billabong with a simple grounding exercise. This works well with children; it also works well with people who are highly activated and distressed. We use the hand as a focus, bringing our attention to five senses. The reason we choose these five is because they're part of the limbic system, which is the part of your brain that is always awake. It's the part of the brain that controls or takes in information from all of the senses.

### Activity 3.3 The Five Senses

We use the five fingers of the hand as we go through each of the senses. Start with your thumb. Bring your attention to what can you ***smell***. Take a deep breath. What can you smell? Can you smell a coffee? Is someone having lunch? Can you smell the dog? What exactly can you smell? Bring your whole mind and focus only on what you can smell.

Next, your index finger. What can you ***feel*?** Can you feel yourself sitting in the chair? Can you feel your clothes? Are they comfortable? Feel your feet on the earth, on the floor, in your shoes or on the carpet. Bring your senses to what you can feel.

Middle finger: What can you ***taste*?** Just take a moment. Is that the coffee or tea you've been drinking, the chocolates or snacks on the desk? Just bring your senses to what you can taste.

Ring finger. Bring your full attention to what you can ***hear***. If it's easier, close your eyes for this. Can you hear the clock? Can you hear the dog barking? Can you hear yourself breathing? Can you hear other people giggling in the room? What can you hear?

Little finger. Now open your eyes. What can you ***see***? Bring your full attention to what you can see. Look around, find something to look at. Is it bright? Is it dark in the room? Really bring your mind to what you can see.

Okay so now you've grounded yourself by bringing your frontal lobes and your limbic system together. All those thoughts, all those worries, all that other business has been set aside so you can focus on the here and now.

What you have just done can be recognised as a *sensory-motor* exercise.

### Activity 3.4 Check-out and Reflection

These beautiful stones (Fig. 3.3) are individual pieces of artwork by Donna Hensen, the Aboriginal artist we work with. We often offer the stones as gifts to people who do our face-to-face training.

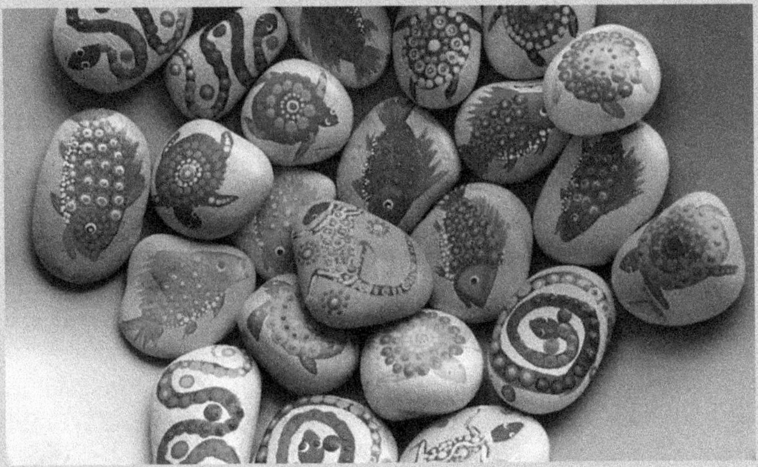

**Fig. 3.3** Painted stones. Source: Photo taken at one of our trainings

Take a moment to check in with your body. What are you feeling? See if you can identify where in your body you are feeling it.

Then consider these reflective questions:

- How much do you know about your own culture and heritage?
- What aspects of your cultural perspective do you think you need to be conscious of when you interact with people from another culture?
- Think about a time when you met or worked with a person who had a different cultural perspective from yours. What values or beliefs of yours were challenged? What would you do differently now you have more understanding of cultural safety?
- What were your first reactions when you saw the photo from Gaua Island?
- Knowing the whole story, how do you see it now?

## References and Further Reading

Belfrage, M. (2007). Why "culturally safe" health care? *Medical Journal of Australia, 186*(10), 537–538. https://doi.org/10.5694/j.1326-5377.2007.tb01032.x

Bennett, B., & Gates, T. G. (2019). Teaching cultural humility for social workers serving LGBTQI Aboriginal communities in Australia. *Social Work Education, 38*(5), 604–617. https://doi.org/10.1080/02615479.2019.1588872

Bennett, B., Zubrzycki, J., & Bacon, V. (2011). What do we know? The experiences of social workers working alongside Aboriginal people. *Australian Social Work, 64*(1), 20–37. https://doi.org/10.1080/0312407X.2010.511677

Bennett, B., Redfern, H., & Zubrzycki, J. (2018). Cultural responsiveness in action: Co-constructing social work curriculum resources with Aboriginal communities. *British Journal of Social Work, 48*(3), 808–825.

Brascoupé, S., & Waters, C. (2009). Cultural safety: Exploring the applicability of the concept of cultural safety to aboriginal health and community wellness. *International Journal of Indigenous Health, 5*(2), 6–41.

Browne, A. J., & Varcoe, C. (2006). Critical cultural perspectives and health care involving Aboriginal peoples. *Contemporary Nurse, 22*(2), 155–168. https://doi.org/10.5172/conu.2006.22.2.155

Burchum, J. L. R. (2002). Cultural competence: An evolutionary perspective. *Nursing Forum, 37*(4), 5–15. https://doi.org/10.1111/j.1744-6198.2002.tb01287.x

Campinha-Bacote, J. (2019). Cultural competemility: A paradigm shift in the cultural competence versus cultural humility debate – Part I. *OJIN: The Online Journal of Issues in Nursing, 24*(1). https://doi.org/10.3912/OJIN.Vol24No01PPT20

Curtis, E., Jones, R., Tipene-Leach, D., Walker, C., Loring, B., Paine, S.-J., & Reid, P. (2019). Why cultural safety rather than cultural competency is required to achieve health equity: A literature review and recommended definition. *International Journal for Equity in Health, 18*(174), 1–17. https://doi.org/10.1186/s12939-019-1082-3

Daniels-Mayes, S. (2019). A courageous conversation with racism: Revealing the racialised stories of Aboriginal deficit for pre-service teachers. *The Australian Educational Researcher, 47*, 537–554. https://doi.org/10.1007/s13384-019-00360-0

Danso, R. (2018). Cultural competence and cultural humility: A critical reflection on key cultural diversity concepts. *Journal of Social Work, 18*(4), 410–430. https://doi.org/10.1177/1468017316654341

Downing, R., Kowal, E., & Paradies, Y. (2011). Indigenous cultural training for health workers in Australia. *International Journal for Quality in Health Care, 23*(3), 247–257. https://doi.org/10.1093/intqhc/mzr008

Durey, A., Wynaden, D., & O'Kane, M. (2014). Improving forensic mental health care to indigenous Australians: Theorizing the intercultural space. *Journal of Psychiatric and Mental Health Nursing, 21*(4), 296–302. https://doi.org/10.1111/jpm.12105

Edwards, J. B. (2016). Cultural intelligence for clinical social work practice. *Clinical Social Work Journal, 44*(3), 211–220. https://doi.org/10.1007/s10615-015-0543-4

Farrelly, T., & Lumby, B. (2009). A best practice approach to cultural competence training. *Aboriginal and Islander Health Worker Journal, 33*(5), 14–22.

Fernando, T., & Bennett, B. (2018). Creating a culturally safe space when teaching Aboriginal content in social work: A scoping review. *Australian Social Work, 72*(1), 47–61. https://doi.org/10.1080/0312407x.2018.1518467

Fisher-Borne, M., Cain, J. M., & Martin, S. L. (2015). From mastery to accountability: Cultural humility as an alternative to cultural competence. *Social Work Education, 34*(2), 165–181. https://doi.org/10.1080/02615479.2014.977244

Foronda, C., Baptiste, D.-L., Reinholdt, M. M., & Ousman, K. (2016). Cultural humility: A concept analysis. *Journal of Transcultural Nursing, 27*(3), 210–217. https://doi.org/10.1177/1043659615592677

Fredericks, B. (2008). The need to extend beyond the knowledge gained in cross-cultural awareness training. *The Australian Journal of Indigenous Education, 37*(S1), 81–89.

Funston, L. (2013). Aboriginal and Torres Strait Islander worldviews and cultural safety transforming sexual assault service provision for children and young people. *International Journal of Environmental Research and Public Health, 10*(9), 3818–3833. https://doi.org/10.3390/ijerph10093818

Gollan, S., & Stacey, K. (2021). *Australian evaluation society first nations cultural safety framework*. Australian Evaluation Society.

Halloran, M. (2004). Cultural maintenance and trauma in Indigenous Australia. *Elaw Journal: Murdoch University Electronic Journal of Law, 11*(4), 1–12.

Hamilton, F. (n.d.). *Creating culturally safe spaces*. Retrieved from http://www.utsdesignindex.com/researchmethod/culturally-safe-spaces/

Harris, T., & O'Donoghue, K. (2020). Developing culturally responsive supervision through Yarn Up Time and the CASE supervision model. *Australian Social Work, 73*(1), 64–76. https://doi.org/10.1080/0312407X.2019.1658796

Herring, S., Spangaro, J., Lauw, M., & McNamara, L. (2013). The intersection of trauma, racism, and cultural competence in effective work with Aboriginal people: Waiting for trust. *Australian Social Work, 66*(1), 104–117. https://doi.org/10.1080/0312407x.2012.697566

Laverty, M., McDermott, D. R., & Calma, T. (2017). Embedding cultural safety in Australia's main health care standards. *The Medical Journal of Australia, 207*(1), 15–16.

Mackean, T., Fisher, M., Friel, S., & Baum, F. (2020). A framework to assess cultural safety in Australian public policy. *Health Promotion International, 35*(2), 340–351. https://doi.org/10.1093/heapro/daz011

McCall, J., & Lauridsen-Hoegh, P. (2014). Trauma and cultural safety: Providing quality care to HIV-infected women of Aboriginal descent. *The Journal of the Association of Nurses in AIDS Care, 25*(1), S70–S78. https://doi.org/10.1016/j.jana.2013.05.005

McGough, S., Wynaden, D., & Wright, M. (2018). Experience of providing cultural safety in mental health to Aboriginal patients: A grounded theory study. *International Journal of Mental Health Nursing, 27*(1), 204–213. https://doi.org/10.1111/inm.12310

Nummenmaa, L., Glerean, E., Hari, R., & Hietanen, J. K. (2014). Bodily maps of emotions. *Proceedings of the National Academy of Sciences, 111*(2), 646–651. https://doi.org/10.1073/pnas.1321664111

Ortega, R., & Faller, K. (2011). Training child welfare workers from an intersectional cultural humility perspective: A paradigm shift. *Child Welfare, 90*(5), 27–49. Retrieved from https://ezproxy.scu.edu.au/login?url=https://search.ebscohost.com/login.aspx?direct=true&db=mnh&AN=EPTOC104543682&site=ehost-live

Papps, E., & Ramsden, I. (1996). Cultural safety in nursing: The New Zealand experience. *International Journal of Quality Health Care, 8*(5), 491–497.

Phillips, G. L. (2015). *Dancing with power: Aboriginal health, cultural safety and medical education.* (PhD), Monash University, Melbourne.

Ramsden, I. (1992). *Kawa Whakaruruhau: Guidelines for Nursing and Midwifery Education.* Nursing Council of New Zealand.

Ramsden, I. (2002). *Cultural safety and nursing education in Aotearoa and Te Waipounamu* (PhD). Victoria University of Wellington, Wellington.

Reyes Cruz, M., & Sonn, C. C. (2011). (De) colonizing culture in community psychology: Reflections from critical social science. *American Journal of Community Psychology, 47*(1-2), 203–214.

Rosen, D., McCall, J., & Goodkind, S. (2017). Teaching critical self-reflection through the lens of cultural humility: An assignment in a social work diversity course. *Social Work Education, 36*(3), 289–298. https://doi.org/10.1080/02615479.2017.1287260

Secombe, P. J., Brown, A., Bailey, M. J., & Pilcher, D. (2019). Equity for indigenous Australians in intensive care. *Medical Journal of Australia, 211*(7), 297–299. https://doi.org/10.5694/mja2.50339

Smith, K., Fatima, Y., & Knight, S. (2017). Are primary healthcare services culturally appropriate for Aboriginal people? Findings from a remote community. *Australian Journal of Primary Health, 23*(3), 236–242. https://doi.org/10.1071/PY16110

Te, M., Blackstock, F., & Chipchase, L. (2019). Fostering cultural responsiveness in physiotherapy: Curricula survey of Australian and Aotearoa New Zealand physiotherapy programs. *BMC Medical Education, 19*(1), 1–12.

Tervalon, M., & Murray-Garcia, J. (1998). Cultural humility versus cultural competence: A critical distinction in defining physician training outcomes in multicultural education. *Journal of Health Care for the Poor and Underserved, 9*(2), 117–125. https://doi.org/10.1353/hpu.2010.0233

Thomson, N. (2005). Cultural respect and related concepts: A brief summary of the literature. *Australian Indigenous Health Bulletin, 5*(4), 1–11.

Tujague, N., & Ryan, K. (2021). Ticking the box of 'cultural safety' is not enough: Why trauma-informed practice is critical to Indigenous healing. *Rural and Remote Health, 21*(3). https://doi.org/10.22605/RRH6411

Varcoe, C., Browne, A. J., Ford-Gilboe, M., Dion Stout, M., McKenzie, H., Price, R., Bungay, V., Smye, V., Inyallie, J., & Day, L. (2017). Reclaiming our spirits: Development and pilot testing of a health promotion intervention for Indigenous women who have experienced intimate partner violence. *Research in Nursing & Health, 40*(3), 237–254.

# 4

# Yarning at the Campsite: Understanding Trauma

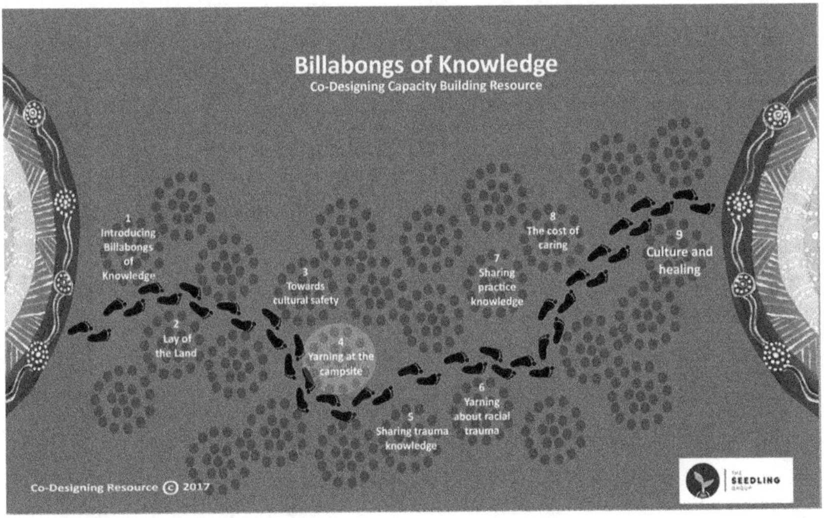


I acknowledge the Aboriginal and Torres Strait Islander Peoples as the original Australians and recognise them as the traditional custodians of knowledge for these lands. I do not live on my country today, but on the lands for the Ngunnawal and Ngambri People of the Canberra region, and I offer my respect and thanks to them for that privilege. I pay my respects to Elders, the holders of knowledge for these lands, both those past, those who lead us today and to those that will guide us in the future. I honour

 
N. Tujague, K. Ryan, *Cultural Safety in Trauma-Informed Practice from a First Nations Perspective*, https://doi.org/10.1007/978-3-031-13138-7_4

their enduring connections to the land, the waters and the sky, and to culture. I also acknowledge those who have been taken, who have had their connections to their People and their Country stolen from them, and I pay my respects to their loss, to their resilience, and to their sorrow.
Belinda Gibb, proud Dharug woman

## Introduction

At the previous billabong we finished by talking about the first principle of trauma work, cultural safety. We discussed how cultural safety is only possible if cultural worldviews are understood and respected when supporting healing work and integrated therapeutic responses (O'Brien, 2010). At this billabong we unpack what trauma is. We look at trauma in the brain, the neuroscience of trauma and trauma in the body. We explore how we work with trauma in Aboriginal and Torres Strait Islander contexts. We talk about how trauma affects us on a systems level and discuss fight, flight, freeze and befriend as types of threat response. We touch on 'polyvagal theory', which casts light on the essential role the vagus nerve plays in the body. We conclude by examining Attachment Theory and the impact of early traumatic experiences through findings from the ACE Study.

But before we start, let's take a moment to connect mind and body.

**Activity 4.1 Guided Body Scan and Check-in**

This is a focused relaxation and mindfulness tool.

Find a seat, get yourself comfortable and put your feet on the ground. If you're in a brightly lit room, turn the lights down low. If you have some essential oils you can burn, even better. Close your eyes for a moment.

Think about your feet. Are they relaxed? Kick your shoes off if you want to and if it's cold where you are, you might want to put on some thick socks. Feel the soles of your feet and imagine for a moment there are roots growing out of the soles of your feet. Feel them pushing their way through the floor, through the concrete slab into the ground and into the earth. They're pushing all the way down to the water table, where they get sustenance as you sit and relax. Wriggle your toes a little bit and then relax your toes. Relax your feet, relax your ankles, relax your calves. Let your knees just fall out slightly and relax those major muscle groups in your thighs. Let yourself sink into the chair. Let your hips relax.

(*continued*)

**Activity 4.1 (continued)**

Think for a moment what's going on in your tummy. Just appreciate that feeling and then let it go and relax. Take a deep breath in and relax your chest. Gently draw your shoulders away from your ears and relax your shoulders. Move your fingers a little bit, throw away any tension in them. Relax your fingers and put your hands on your lap. Let your arms grow heavy, relax your back and your neck. Relax your jaw. Relax your cheeks and let your eyelids get heavy. Smooth those corrugator muscles between your eyebrows. Relax your scalp.

Now imagine there's a string tied to the crown of your head, and someone is gently pulling that string. It stretches your head and all your vertebrae upwards. Your blood rushes in and renews your whole nervous system. As you pull your head up, your chin tucks in, your tummy tucks in. Now, take a big breath in, and a long breath out. Big breath in, long breath out. Okay. When you're ready, just open your eyes. Move everything a little bit and come back to the room where you are.

How do you feel? Where do you feel it in your body? What feeling word would you use to describe it?

## Circles of Knowledge and Connection

We have designed the Circles of Knowledge and Connection Model (Fig. 4.1) as a case formulation tool that you can use with your clients. This model[1] represents the way Aboriginal and Torres Strait Islander knowledge is connected to all parts of social and emotional wellbeing. The red relates to our thoughts, beliefs, spirit and spirituality; the blue to our connection to Country, community, family and kinship; the yellow to our physical being; and the green to our ancestors, our culture or our roots. It is a simple representation of what practitioners call 'holistic case formulation', where we look at the whole of the person. We understand that all our behaviours or thoughts are being influenced by the whole of the context that we live in. This case formulation 'map' is a symbolic representation of the SEWB Wheel we talked about in Chap. 2.

[1] Watch https://vimeo.com/user131141829/review/508691254/fe6073aeed for Kelleigh's demonstration of how she uses an earlier version of this model.

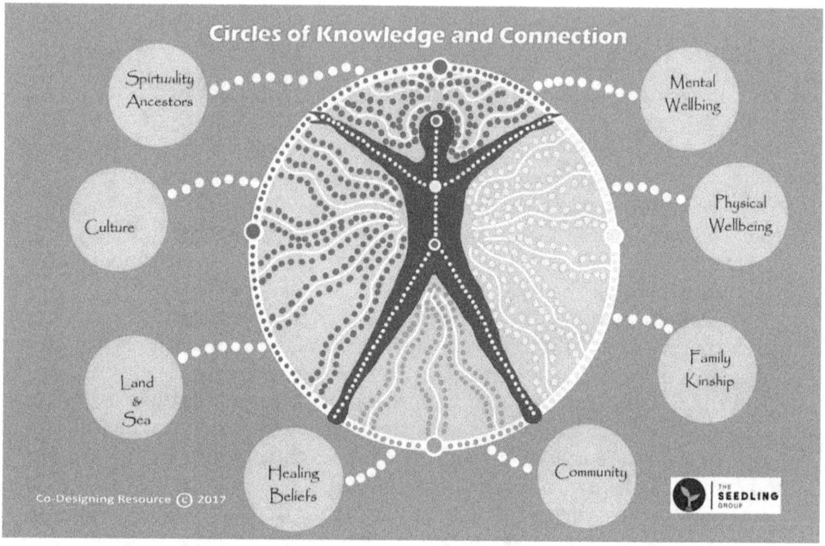


**Fig. 4.1** Circles of knowledge and connection. Source: © The Seedling Group; artwork Donna Hensen

We find this model useful for two reasons. First, it's very clear and makes sense to Aboriginal and Torres Strait Islander Peoples, our 'mob'. The model uses symbols that are significant to collective communities in Australia. It shows the connecting lines outside of the circle, representing connection/travel between places or concepts. We call it the 'Circle of Knowledge' because it's about understanding what's going on for your client *and* what's going on for you, giving you a much better idea of how you can help identify all of the elements of social and emotional wellbeing. This situates you as practitioner *within* the relationship with your client, not separate from it.

The second reason is that this model embeds the '8-ways of learning' (Yunkaporta & Kirby, 2011; Yunkaporta & McGinty, 2009) that we talked about in Chap. 2.

*Kelleigh: The whole thing is a learning map for both of us. Its non-linear so the client can say what's important to them and where they want to go next in their healing journey. Its non-verbal to get past any language or literacy issues, allowing description through symbols and sharing stories about community and land links in those symbols that we draw. Then together we deconstruct and reconstruct injury and meaning for healing.*

It provides an opportunity for an individual to self-reflect and name what is of importance to them, things which might never be discussed in a biomedical, individualist practice model.

## What Is Trauma?

Trauma has been defined as the symptoms or behavioural changes left after someone has faced an event they perceive to be life threatening (Herman, 2015; Van der Kolk, 2015), meaning it is overwhelming or beyond the individual's ability to continue to function normally. It changes the way we feel, not only about our ability to feel safe and in control, but also how we form connections. What this implies is that a traumatic event that is beyond your body's nervous system's resources to cope, leaves changes in the nervous system that, unless healed, will continue to be on the lookout for danger. The event itself can be physical, psychological, environmental or spiritual; it can be experienced accumulatively, collectively or individually. Robin Shapiro (2010, 2020) explains trauma as an experience that overwhelms our ability to cope and leaves our relationships and our brains with the challenge of finding a way to integrate and function well. Trauma is thus not defined in terms of the original event itself, but in terms of the *body's ability to respond with the resources it has available to it.* It is influenced by both intergenerational elements and lived experiences.

Trauma is *subjective* in the sense that it activates the body's primal threat fear system of *befriend, fight, flight or freeze,* that we examine in more detail later in the chapter. Once trauma pushes a person beyond their normal resources to cope, it changes the way that person responds to the same stimulus or similar stimuli forever. What happens is the trauma presents your brain with the challenge to find a way to integrate this new traumatic threat response into our normal, everyday living. If the threat was one your nervous system could cope with normally, it would just go ahead and respond, calm itself, make sense of it, integrate the experience into your knowledge system and record this to deal with future events. This is what we call 'resilience'.

To illustrate, let's say you and I are both in a car accident together. We both experienced the same event. However, you might get a fright, but be able to resume your normal functioning in a few days. Whereas I might have nightmares. I might become hypervigilant. I might even stop driving, fearful that it's going to happen again. Both of our threat responses have been activated, but you managed to extinguish the fear response, integrate the event into your long-term memory, contextualise it and move on. However, for some reason, I have not. It continues to interfere with my normal functioning.

***Nicole:*** *The way I like to think about the differences between how we respond to events, is you go through childhood having lots of bust-ups, grazing your knee, that sort of stuff, but things heal over. I think of these as just hurts that happen; they heal completely and you forget about them. But the trauma or 'scar', is something that changes you forever.*

*I have a story from when I was young that illustrates this. On the inside left of my shin, I have this tiny little scar. I was about eight years old and I still remember the day I got that scar. We were living in Woorabinda, and mum and us kids were all in the front yard saying goodbye to visitors. On our fence was a piece of timber with rows of barbed wire underneath the timber. I remember I was walking up on the fence, something I wasn't allowed to do. Mum was distracted and I was doing a sort of a balancing act on the timber on top of the fence. I slipped and fell over. A piece of the barbed wire underneath hooked into my leg. I was hanging up by that piece of barbed wire. That's how I remember it. I remember mum, I remember what happened, I remember that feeling. I remember everyone rushing around. I remember the front yard.*

*Because of that enduring memory it was more than a hurt; it was a trauma. Because I still have that scar, it changed me. It changed the sense I had at that age that I was indestructible. For me, that's the difference between a hurt that heals over and a trauma that changes the way you see the world or changes you forever. When I think back to that incident, it has stayed in my whole body and mind and changed the way I live in the world.*

## The DSM Definition of Trauma

Simply put, the DSM (which stands for *Diagnostic Statistical Manual of Mental Disorders*) is a manual used by health professionals which gives us straightforward tools to standardise clusters of symptoms that are present in our client in different contexts over a period of time. This guides us to make a diagnosis. Psychologists who use it, like to refer to the DSM as a 'living document', meaning that every few years we make changes to the manual as we learn new things as more research is published. The DSM-5 (published in 2013) is the most recent edition at time of writing this book. It made a number of changes to the definition of trauma from the DSM-IV (originally published in 2000). The current DSM-5 definition of trauma requires "actual or threatened death, serious injury, or sexual violence" (*American Psychiatric Association*, 2013, p. 271). Stressful events not involving an immediate threat to life or physical injury such as psychosocial stressors (e.g., divorce or job loss) are not considered trauma in this definition (Pai et al., 2017; Jones & Cureton, 2014).

## First Nations Peoples and the DSM

One of the main limitations of the DSM is that it is not 'normed' on First Nations Peoples (Overmars, 2010) or people who belong to collective cultures. Nor does it apply to people in developing nations that do not have the resources to support research. Much of the research testing is done with non-Indigenous, middle-class university graduates, or people from non-Indigenous and individualistic cultures who are available to do surveys or clinical trials. Things like your spirituality or your connection to Country aren't taken into account, or recognised as having an influence, because they're not part of individualist cultures normed in research.

When we work in Aboriginal and Torres Strait Islander communities and start talking about the DSM, we often ask, "what can you recognise that is missing from the DSM definitions?" What becomes obvious from their responses is that when we look at that holistic model of health, the SEWB Wheel, the DSM completely disregards the spiritual, ancestral and connection to Country elements of health and wellbeing.

***Kelleigh**: As a practitioner who works with First Nations Peoples, I still find the DSM a helpful tool when someone presents with very complex symptoms. I'll collect information and ask questions about whether they are seeing signs and behaviours of those symptoms at home, or at work or at school. If they are, I ask about what's happening at the time when those symptoms are presenting. You might want to understand the difference between a depressive episode and post-traumatic stress disorder (PTSD). You would look at the manual to find out what the cluster of symptoms is telling you. It doesn't mean that if I see five out of the eleven symptoms that I make a diagnosis. What it means is that I'm aware that my client has symptoms that are present in the criteria for a particular diagnosis. But I also know that my client's neuropsychological responses are expressed through behaviours that are trying to protect them and communicate something. They have an intent, just as all behaviours are driven by intent. As I look through a cultural lens in my practice, I focus on exploring the meaning of the intent behind the presenting behaviours.*

We might instead use the term 'symptomology'. You are more likely to hear health professionals say things like 'symptoms of bipolar disorder' or 'symptoms of schizophrenia', instead of making a direct diagnosis of bipolar or schizophrenia or using those kinds of labels. We need to be careful about labelling people who present with particular symptoms too quickly. Before the age of 18, it's not helpful to give a child a label, because they are still developing. We will say they have 'behaviours of …', or they 'have symptoms of …', or they might be 'having an episode', but we avoid labelling them because of the stigma attached to mental illness. On the other hand, labelling could be important if the client needs some specialised professional help. For example, if your client is a child who has some very specific behaviours and needs, then knowing what you're dealing with and knowing whether you need to call in an occupational therapist, a speech pathologist or someone else who can help, can make a real difference to your client's treatment.

Often when people are experiencing painful, problematic behaviour and when they get a diagnosis, suddenly, it's a relief: "oh, so it's not me. I totally get it. I get that this is a thing". And if you know what's wrong, it's like any fear, when you know what it is, you can address it. If I say to a client who fears they are going mad: "actually, your symptoms sound like mild depression. It normally lasts for this long and these strategies can help. Depression hates exercise, so get some exercise, do some laughing …". But if someone has a major depressive disorder, saying those things might help, but there are other things that may make a bigger difference. Once we recognise that the problematic behaviours are present all the time, telling the client to do something without getting any assistance may not be useful.

If you say "just reach out" to someone who is seriously depressed or has a major depressive disorder, reaching out may not be something they are capable of. It becomes a form of 'blaming the victim'. This is why culturally, *outreach* services are more effective. We who provide the service are the ones who reach out, because we shouldn't always expect the person who's unwell to be able to ask for help. That's one fundamental difference between non-Indigenous and Indigenous practices. We facilitate reaching out, we go to them; we don't ask them to spend the money on coming to us instead of buying food. We often go to them *with food,* as part of our reciprocal practice.

## Trauma and Neuroscience

How the therapeutic community thinks about trauma has changed radically with changes in technology. Up until the 1980s, trauma was mostly talked about in terms of a physical injury of some kind. Then along came technologies like Magnetic Resonance Imaging (MRI) machines, equipment that enabled us to see what was happening in the brain and in different organs in the body following a traumatic event. This helped us understand that beyond physical trauma, psychological trauma sets off physiological processes as well (Evans & Coccoma, 2014).

What Elders and traditional healers have always known can now be shown in visual representations because of the advances in neuroscience. Once neuroscience linked what was happening in the body *and* in the brain, we could see that some behaviours were clearly associated with psychological trauma. Suddenly, when a patient presented with problems like recurring headaches, stomach problems, feeling anxious, scared or angry all the time, it was possible to see what was happening in their brain. This meant that the disciplines that study human behaviour (psychology and psychiatry) and the discipline of medicine had to come together to explain and to work on those problems. While this led to more collaboration between the disciplines, the hierarchical nature of professions still produces some tension about whose knowledge about trauma is more important or takes precedence.

Despite these recent developments and changes, psychological trauma is still the 'elephant in the room' (Fig. 4.2). We continue to hear doctors and psychiatrists saying: "We didn't study psychological trauma when we were at university. We learned about schizophrenia and bipolar disorder (BPD), but we didn't actually go into psychological trauma and how it affects the body's anatomy and physiology". It is still possible to be dealing with members of the medical profession who didn't learn the about the effects of psychological trauma until after their basic university training. That's challenging when you're trying to get medical help for a client or for yourself.

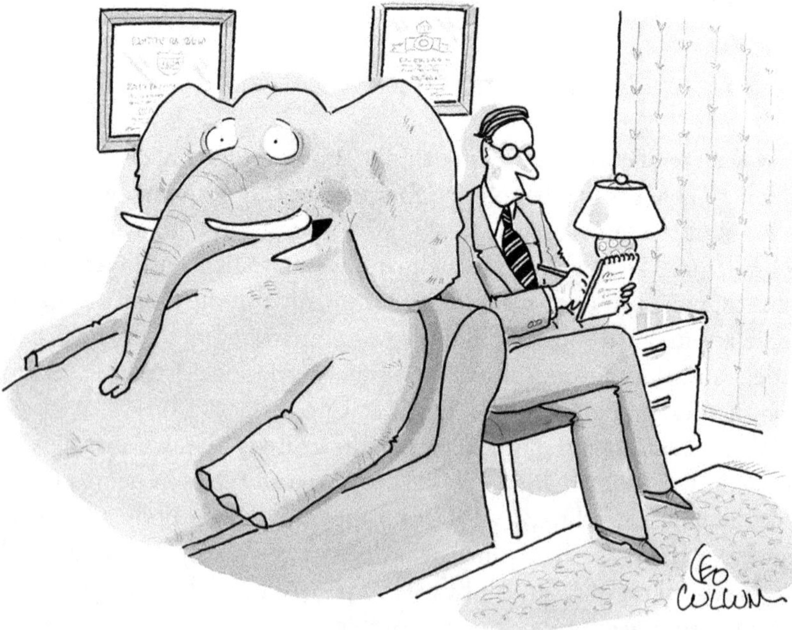

*"I'm right there in the room, and no one even acknowledges me."*

**Fig. 4.2** Elephant in the room. Source: *New Yorker* magazine (2006) Volume 18

## Structure of the Brain

In order to understand how trauma impacts on the brain, we offer a couple of simple models that help explain the main structures in the brain that we refer to throughout the book.

## A Simple Model of Brain Structure: The 'Triune Brain' (Fig. 4.3)

The 'triune brain' model (Maclean, 1990; Ploog, 2003; Sweeton, 2019) describes the three basic parts of the whole brain in terms of the **survival** brain, the **emotional** brain and the **thinking** brain. While this is a highly simplified explanation of brain activity and organisation, this model is useful because it provides an easy-to-understand approximation of the hierarchy of brain functions. It's also a good way to understand brain

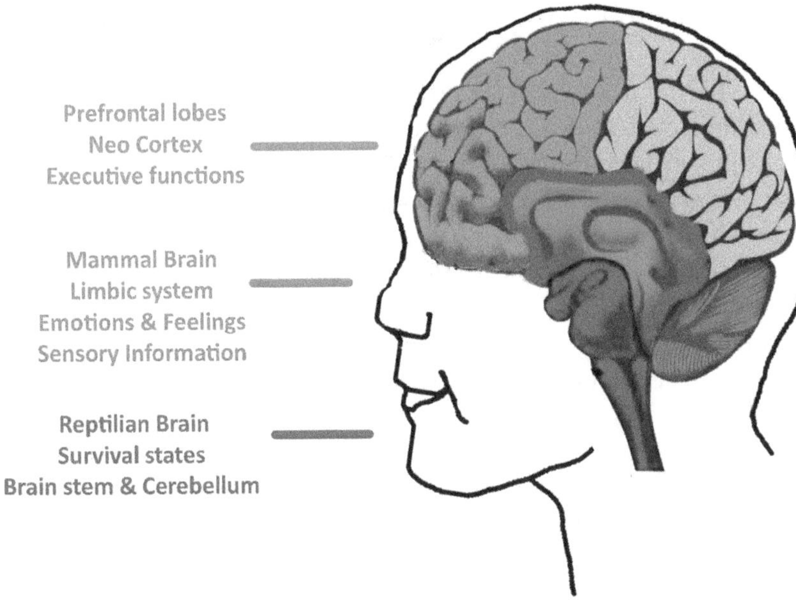


**Fig. 4.3** The Triune Brain. Source: The Triune Brain © The Seedling Group 2022; artwork by Donna Hensen

activation and the reasoning behind the time it takes for your thinking brain to come online. We should note here that the triune brain fell out of favour because of a misconception that the model implied the three parts of the brain operated independently of each other.

The **survival brain** (or the reptilian brain) sits in the brainstem and is thought to be the first part of the brain to develop in the process of evolution (Cozolino, 2017; Schoenemann, 2006). It's the part of the brain that is continually switched on, always searching for danger. Its job is to keep us alive. In the red zone, the survival brain is taking in all the information from the world around us. We're always seeing, smelling, hearing, feeling, touching; we're always taking in information and sorting it.

For example, you're sitting reading a book, totally engrossed in the story, having a good time. Then someone comes up behind you. Even if you can't see that person, you sense that someone is there. Your frontal cortex (the thinking brain) can be still reading the story and taking in the storyline, but your whole body is aware that someone's there; your reptilian brain is picking up on potential danger in the room.

The second part of the brain in this model is called the **emotional brain** (or the mammalian brain) where your limbic system lives. It is responsible for all sensory information and emotional processing. It makes memories made from the stimuli that is taken in. An example: I was eating my favourite chicken curry and got food poisoning; now every time I smell curry or see that restaurant, I feel anxious.

The **thinking brain**, or the neocortex or frontal cortex is the part of the brain that says: "I'm not acting rationally, not all chicken curry is going to make me sick". This is the reasoning part of your brain, the logical, strategic part of your brain in action. But if you're operating out of your limbic or emotional brain, you just don't listen to that calm, sensible, reasoning brain.

The last part of the brain that comes online here is your thinking brain, your upper brain, the frontal or neocortex. That part takes 24 milliseconds to come to the party, while your reptilian brain only takes 12 milliseconds (Evans & Coccoma, 2014). An example might be: I'm walking along a path and I look down and see a snake. My reptilian brain registers "danger, alert, stop, run, do whatever you can to get away". I'm already responding from my survival brain and getting ready to act. But then I look again and see "oh, it's only a stick, it's not actually a snake". That's because my thinking brain has kicked in. My neocortex reasoning says: "if it was a snake, it would be moving now. It's not moving now, I don't need to get out of the way, it's only a stick."

## Model of Brain Structure with Amygdala and Hippocampus (Fig. 4.4)

This more detailed model shows us important parts of the brain, like the amygdala and the hippocampus, that come into play when there's a threat. Those cogs going up the neck represent all that incoming information, travelling up the spinal cord, first entering the reptilian brain

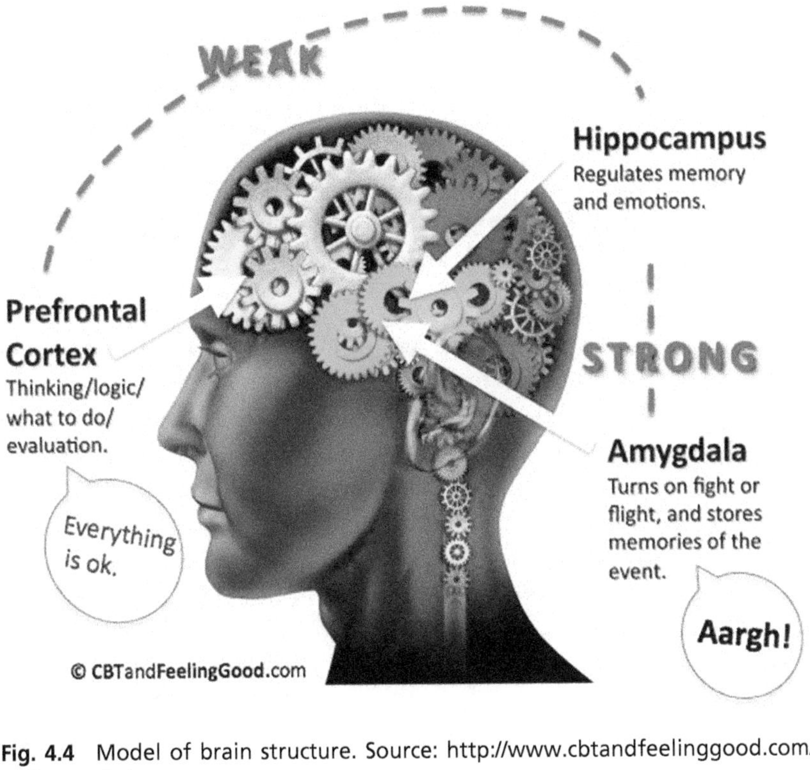


Fig. 4.4 Model of brain structure. Source: http://www.cbtandfeelinggood.com/ with permission

through the brain stem or 'base brain'. In the 'midbrain' (the green cogs) the information from the base brain combines with the emotions or feelings attached to that information from the emotional brain.

The amygdala is basically your brain's alarm system. It's the part that responds, "okay, I'm taking in information, there's something up ahead that looks like a snake or it could be a stick". It sends out the alarm. As neurochemicals are activated, the amygdala sets off the alarm and checks in with your hippocampus.

***Nicole**: I like to think of the hippocampus as like a big hippopotamus, because he looks like he would be able to store a lot of memories.*

The hippocampus, embedded deep inside your brain, is one of the first parts of you that starts to form and grow. As it is one of the oldest parts, *it remembers everything*. While the amygdala is your alarm system, the hippocampus is your 'hippo' full of information made from all those connections and memories.

The job of your prefrontal cortex, your 'frontal lobes' (the yellow cogs), is to work things out, to problem solve. *It is less active when you are facing a threat.*

## Responses to Threat: Befriend, Fight, Flight or Freeze

Befriend, fight, flight and freeze are all examples *of threat activation.*[2] Those responses are a good thing because they are what keep humans and other species alive. While people often assume that these threat or stress responses are types of trauma, they are actually the way your body *responds* when it senses danger or threat. When we go into one or more of these threat responses, it's our body's way of preparing us to survive the danger.

Problems arise when these responses become habitual and are not always an activation in response to a direct threat. For example, someone who's habitually aggressive could be stuck in **fight** mode. Somebody who is not able to settle down in one place, always wandering from place to

[2] The idea of 'fight or flight' was first introduced by Walter Cannon in 1914 (Cannon, 1914) after observing the behaviour of mice in stressful situations.

place or relationship to relationship, could be stuck in **flight** mode. Extreme risk-taking behaviour can also be another type of flight, as can personal confusion (Sheehan, 2012). When we see these types of behaviour, we don't often recognise them as types of hyper-arousal. *Hyper*-arousal is a term used for that type of activation when the body is going into fight or flight.

The **freeze** response can look like someone who is not responding, feeling nothing, being unable to move or fight back, feeling hopeless or depressed, or even having a sedentary lifestyle. When people self-harm, that can be like a freeze response. Some describe freeze as similar to having the accelerator on full speed and the brake flat to the floor at the same time (Roelofs, 2017). You're not going anywhere. But it doesn't mean that all that petrol isn't pouring into the engine and all those revs aren't roaring. The term for that type of activation, where the person is stuck, passive or 'frozen', is *hypo*-arousal.

While you are probably familiar with the terms 'fight, flight or freeze', psychologists have proposed another response to threat or stress that you may not have come across, that of '**tend and befriend**'. This was originally thought to be a more likely response in females. 'Tending' involves the woman taking care of herself and her children to 'promote safety and reduce stress' (Taylor, et al., 2000, p. 411), while 'befriending' involves building and maintaining social networks to reinforce protection. A good example of tending and befriending behaviour is in the 2015 movie *Room*, based on the book by Irish Canadian author Emma Donoghue (Donoghue, 2010). A more recent study (Levy et al., 2019) argues that both men and women can engage in tend and befriend behaviours, and it is their individual 'attachment style' that will determine whether they are more likely to choose fight/flight or tend/befriend, rather than their gender. For First Nations people, we sometimes see 'befriending' as an act of survival, like the Aboriginal worker who finds herself making excuses for a non-Indigenous co-worker who makes racist comments, because making a scene could risk her losing her job.

***Nicole***: *I feel that I naturally go to freeze, rather than fight or flight. If I'm in bed in the middle of the night and I hear a sound in the house, I'm the one that freezes in my bed. I'm hoping they take everything they want and then leave. Whereas Kelleigh naturally goes to fight. She looks for something to hit them with and goes looking for them.*

When you're in your fear response, whether it's befriend, fight, flight or freeze, your reptilian brain tells you, "there's danger, there's danger" and you stay in that hyper- or hypo-aroused state. Staying in that state is exhausting because your body is designed to go into befriend, fight, flight or freeze to save you; it's designed to go to that state only in short bursts. Our bodies are not *made* to be in that type of activation all the time. That threat response is all about saving you from immediate danger at one point in time.

Every day in our modern lives we have stresses. The more stress you have without coming back to balance, the more likely your body will stay in that stress response state. This means that for many First Nations Peoples the ongoing stress we live with everyday such as being removed from Country, racial trauma or financial instability, adds a whole lot more activation to an already activated nervous system. We start defining people as having a 'behaviour problem' or having a 'problematic personality', when in reality they could be in a permanent state of response activation, like fight or flight. They're removing themselves, or they're angry all the time, or they're always late or they can't pay attention. This could be because they're attending to other information coming in. When we are working with people who are in these persistent hyper- or hypo-aroused states, we need to consider everything else that's going on in their lives.

## Window of Tolerance

The idea of a 'Window of Tolerance', a state of optimal arousal, was first introduced by psychiatrist Dan Siegel (1999). This model (Fig. 4.5), based on Siegel's concept, is a helpful way to illustrate what we've been talking about in terms of that fear response. The middle section, the place of 'optimal arousal' is when the two systems are in balance: we're calm, we're relaxed, our neocortex is online, we're thinking, strategising, solving problems and responding appropriately. That's when we are in the Window of Tolerance. When we stay in optimal arousal, we are able to deal appropriately with everyday challenges.

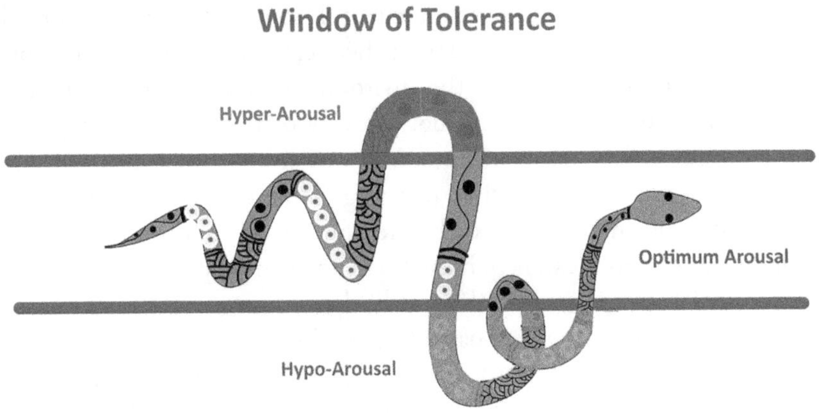


**Fig. 4.5** The Window of Tolerance. Source: The Window of Tolerance © The Seedling Group 2022; artwork Donna Hensen. Adapted from Dan Siegel, 1999

If we have a trauma or some sort of fear response, we can go straight up to **hyper-arousal** (in our adaptation, this is the part of the snake that goes above the top line), where the sympathetic nervous system response has kicked in. When you're in hyper-arousal you'll have symptoms like anxiety, anger, agitation and panic. We also know that your hearing blocks out certain sounds in this state.[3] It pays more attention to the 'threat tones', like raised voices, all that memory it holds of unresolved trauma; all information and sounds outside this tone level are just white noise.

When clients come in hyper-aroused and you start telling them intricate details about something or give them instructions, you can see they're not taking everything you say on board. That's because they're only listening for those things that are going to keep them alive. They are receiving your words, but they're not actually thinking or strategising in the way you expect them to. They are only hearing, using their short-term memory, not integrating the information into meaning or actions, because that requires your frontal lobes, your neocortex, to be available to help out.

If you can see where your client might be sitting in the Window of Tolerance (where they are on the middle part of the snake), that might

[3] https://www.pursuit-of-happiness.org/history-of-happiness/barb-fredrickson/

help you find a way to relate to your client. If someone's in hyper-arousal where their body's being flooded with chemicals like adrenaline and cortisol, it's useful to think about the environment. You can make sure the lights aren't too bright, that it's not a rowdy or busy place, that there's some calmness they can walk into. You can also get them to do some breathing or grounding exercises, bringing their attention to the safety of being with you in this context, before you actually start talking about things. Those actions can help bring them *down* into optimal arousal, the Window of Tolerance, where they are likely to be more receptive.

In **hypo-arousal** (the grey part of the snake that is below the bottom line), we see numbness, shutdown, people not taking care of themselves or losing their boundaries. If your client is in hypo-arousal, they may appear zoned out, flat, non-responsive. You just know they're not with you. You can do things to bring them back *up* into the Window of Tolerance. You could get them to do gentle, straightforward physical actions where they can bring their frontal lobes back online, for instance you could ask: "do you want to make a cup of tea for us while I get our papers ready?" Or you might ask questions where they have to make simple decisions like: "Would you like tea or coffee? Would you like sugar?"

## What Does the Threat Response Look Like in Young Children?

For babies who experience a stressful time while they are still in utero, their nervous systems have already made adjustments by the time they are born. They may cry less, be dissociative or can't settle because they are highly anxious (Perry, 2009; Carrión et al., 2010). These adjustments mean the baby is ready from birth to cope with the environment they are born into. When the child enters early childhood and goes to pre-school, if there's no focused support, these adjustments and behaviours may become reinforced and more established. They may instead be picked up as 'learning difficulties' or 'defiant behaviour', rather than recognised as signs of coping strategies.

In children, the threat response manifests in behaviours. As a *fight* response, some children might imitate the perpetrator, for example, this may manifest as early sexualised behaviour or becoming aggressive towards other students or teachers. A *flight* response might look like withdrawal, avoidance, defiance or distraction, doing what they can to control the situation. For children in *freeze* response, they daydream; they don't want to get out of bed, they don't want to go to school; they don't know how to play. A *befriend* response might be the child who befriends the bully as a way to stay safe, even if the bully treats them badly. If you are a parent or schoolteacher and start seeing some of these behaviours, have a think about where that child could be in the Window of Tolerance and how you might bring them back into that optimal arousal zone. *Only then* can you start to use your familiar teaching techniques with them.

Behind every behaviour is an intent and the intent is to communicate something to you. If you're seeing a child who's acting out, or angry or can't sit still, their behaviour is telling you something. When you look at the Window of Tolerance, ask yourself: "Where are they in terms of their arousal? What could be going on here?" It's probably not that they just don't like the little girl sitting beside them.

***Kelleigh***: *I had a client who used to run away all the time: whenever his parents would take him to school, he'd get out of the window, get out of the door and make a run for it. That's an absolute flight response. When the school put in place mechanisms so he couldn't run, he would just keep himself safe by disconnecting and staying in hypo-arousal. He couldn't interact, he couldn't pay attention, he would daydream. He'd run away emotionally. I could see his body was saying, "I cannot cope with the amount of fear and the drive of that fear that I'm experiencing and you clearly aren't getting it. You clearly can't help me, so I have to help myself."*

This is difficult information for teachers to hear if they haven't studied trauma. Often when we're teaching groups of teachers, they'll say, "so how do we tell the difference between trauma and bad behaviour?" The difficult answer to that is "*there is no such thing as bad behaviour*". It's something we've made up to describe a set of symptoms. There is always something that child is trying to tell you. Remember that the mainstream school system is built on a deficit model of punitive responses to children's behaviour, just like the justice system. It's not holistic; it isn't based on an understanding of trauma.

This is a system that teaches children but doesn't understand the normal responses of a human body, even though the research demonstrating this is robust (Cozolino, 2014, 2017; Evans & Coccoma, 2014; Perry, 2006, 2008). To take that research into account would mean changing the system that works on this punitive model. Even though we know that punishment only brings compliance or defiance, the system is set up to make things work for the teacher. It's good for you as teacher because you'll get through your lesson plan or you'll get through the day, but for that child, they may not actually be learning. In reality, you may be wasting that child's time. If you're being paid to teach, then you may have to ask yourself: "*What more do I need to know to be able to teach here*?"

You can use the Window of Tolerance in your classroom or office for children to show where they feel they are on the snake.

The school system is also merit-driven (we talk in more detail about meritocracy in Chap. 6). The child still stuck in a trauma response not only gets penalised in terms of being embarrassed, considered unintelligent or rebuked for not paying attention or not working hard enough to keep up, when in fact suffering the effects of trauma may make staying engaged near impossible for them. Teaching becomes fear-driven, rather than curiosity-driven.

We can also teach kids to use the Window of Tolerance. When they come into the classroom, they can go up to the Window of Tolerance poster and put a star on where they are, according to how they're feeling. For a teacher, this is gold. If a teacher sees that Jimmy's come in and put a star up in hyper-arousal, she knows that she can give Jimmy something calming to do to start with. If Jimmy comes in and he's in hypo-arousal, he might be the one that takes the mail to the office or some other task that will calm him. Get him out, get him breathing and moving before you expect him to sit down, have his frontal lobes online and problem solve with you. This is what has to happen before he can use all of his brain in the classroom. If you have children in your classroom who are living in traumatic situations or have suffered trauma, then knowing where they are in the Window of Tolerance and when you can start teaching them is critically important.

## The Role of the Autonomic Nervous System

The responses we've been talking about here are very much related to the autonomic nervous system, which is at the core of our threat response. You are probably familiar with the *central* nervous system, our brain, our spinal cord, and all the nerves that go out to our muscles to help us move. Our central nervous system is operating when, for example, we touch a hot plate. Our sensory receptors take messages to our nerves back to our spinal cord; that message goes up to our brain, which says, "that's really hot, and if you don't take your hand away, you're going to end up with blisters." The message goes back down again to your spinal cord, out to your peripheral nerves that innervate your muscles, and get your muscles to pull your hand away. All of that happens in a split second. In fact, in some situations, the message goes back to the spinal cord but doesn't waste time going back to the brain. It makes a decision instantly, in what we call a 'reflex action'.

The autonomic nervous system is one we have very little conscious control over. It's the nervous system that keeps us alive. For instance, it keeps our heart beating. We don't have to consciously think, "I've got to beat my heart. I've got to beat my heart. I've got to beat my heart." Thankfully! That's just something that keeps happening automatically. If it gets very cold outside, the arrector pili muscles in our skin contract, they close up our pores and keep our heat in. We don't have to think, "okay body, keep heat in, it's cold out there." Again, it's something that happens automatically.

The autonomic nervous system is made up of two parts: the *sympathetic* nervous system and the *parasympathetic* nervous system, which each work to keep balance in the body, like a set of scales. When we are faced with danger, our sympathetic nervous system kicks into play with a range of physiological responses. For instance, our pupils dilate, so we can see better. Blood is redirected from all the areas of our body that are not necessary to deal with the threat. For example, if we've just eaten, instead of the blood busily digesting our food, it will leave our stomachs and serve our major muscle groups, those muscles we'll need to either help us fight or run away. When our sympathetic nervous system kicks in, our body also floods with hormones, like adrenaline and cortisol, that give you speed and superhuman strength, like the mother who rushes out and lifts the car the baby is trapped under. We're designed to go into that sympathetic state for short periods of time to get us away from danger, and when the danger has passed, everything comes back into balance.

Imagine you go into a cave and think you see a bear. Your sympathetic nervous system kicks in immediately: your pupils will dilate, your heart will start pumping faster, if your bladder is full, it may even empty itself, you literally 'wet your pants'. Your body gets rid of all the weight it doesn't need to run away or get ready to fight. Then you look again and you think, "oh, it's my old uncle. He was having a snooze and just woke up. It's not a bear at all." Then your parasympathetic nervous system, the opposite side of the scales, kicks in: your heart slows down to its normal rate, all the blood goes back to where it needs to go to start digesting that food, your pupils constrict, and you go back into a state of homeostasis. That's how we're designed to operate every day. We go into fight or flight, we come back down again; we go into fight or flight, we come back down again. For example, we're driving along, someone cuts in front of us, we might go into fight or flight instantly because we've got to brake suddenly. We might want to yell at whoever cuts us off and when no cars are hit and everything is fine, we go back into a state of equilibrium.

This balancing between our sympathetic and parasympathetic nervous systems is what has kept us alive as a species for eons. But it becomes problematic if we are in fight or flight mode constantly. People can be in fight or flight for days, weeks, months, even years, and when that happens, they are stuck in that hyper-aroused state and never get back to equilibrium. When those hormones like cortisol have been pouring down into the body for years on end, like people living in domestic violence situations, children living in situations where there's abuse at home, or people living in a war zone, they can be stuck in a fight, flight or freeze response. This can lead to all sorts of chronic health problems (see Ketheesan et al., 2020 for some of the health problems associated with being in constant states of threat activation).

While most of us are predisposed to one type of threat response, it is possible to change your automatic response depending on what techniques you've learnt to calm yourself or to regulate yourself. However, it is important to remember that one activation to one fight or flight response takes time to re-regulate. It takes about 20 minutes from the time you have a hit of adrenaline to come back to homeostasis if there were no other hits in the meantime.[4] While this might have been possible in previous times, consider how in our everyday lives now our systems are being constantly challenged. You could have a few of those hits just on your drive to work. You may have watched TV and seen horrendous things before you even got out of your house, and that's if you don't have any other challenges during your day. Your system is still trying to rebalance when the next stressful event hits. Add to that worries that simmer in the background, like financial or relationship stresses, and you will have a constantly activated system.

We might be able to calm our nervous system after everyday stresses with good self-care and grounding exercises. With ongoing traumatic stress, this is much more difficult. Some argue that it takes 48 hours for the body to re-balance after a significant stress, like a car accident (Bremner, 2006). When our system can't rebalance itself in time, we don't come back to equilibrium. We stay out of balance and then when another stress hits, we activate from that unbalanced place. So instead of starting from a place of homeostasis, in the Window of Tolerance, where you are nice and calm, with both sympathetic and parasympathetic systems aligned, you have very little space before you are activated by an event that you would otherwise handle calmly. That's what is probably happening when you look at someone the wrong way and they can suddenly go off because they're already super hyper-aroused.

For people who have experienced trauma, their systems can be in constant activation. Apart from the fact that this is very bad for their health, it also means they don't have the resources to seek support to try to rebalance. Remember how your neocortex, your thinking brain, is the first

[4] https://psychcentral.com/blog/anger/2016/06/how-long-does-the-fight-or-flight-reaction-last

one to leave the party when trauma happens? It's also the last one *back* at the party after everything has calmed down. Your thinking brain is the last one to come back online and say, "actually, I've been really stressed, I should probably take some time off," or "I should probably eat some real, nutritious food".

When you're in hyper-arousal or hypo-arousal, a lot of the time you're burning through energy because you're always ready to go. You'll start craving high-energy foods like sugar, chocolate, soft drinks, to get that energy in fast, or fatty foods, like chips, because your body is burning through it. It doesn't need to take time to digest, it doesn't need slow-release energy. It needs high energy, and it needs it *now*. And then we start to see the changes to the way we metabolise sugar. If your stomach is full of chemical because you're under stress, it doesn't matter how much healthy food you eat, you may not be able to absorb the nutrients it contains because it's ready to empty and move on if it needs to (Nirupama, et al., 2018).

## What Do You Do When You Can't Fight Back?

There are certain behavioural signs to look for if someone is stuck outside of the Window of Tolerance, either in hyper- or hypo-arousal. They may feel that there is no way to get rid of that energy or that they can't fight back. These signs include:

- self-destructive behaviour like self-harm, addiction, intoxication or random acts of violence
- a form of 'learned helplessness' (Maier & Seligman, 1976), that conceals their skills and abilities
- inert and calculated disobedience, always waiting to be told to act
- opportunism, theft, fraud, destruction of organisations or property
- jealousy and sabotage
- creating disunity and conflict
- lateral violence (adapted from Sheehan, 2012).

Those behaviours like fighting and drug and alcohol addiction arise from the need to numb the arousal that you can't escape. If you lived in a very racist or volatile environment, home life, or community, a strategy that gives you some time out and allows you to sleep could perhaps be your only escape. But of course, that type of escapism isn't really escaping. Other behaviours that aren't obviously related to a trauma response, such as opportunism, theft, fraud, and destruction of other people's property, are also strategies that can use up that chemical that's driving you, that's keeping you in hyper-arousal. People who are full of rage also feel they are in situations they can't escape, indicating a chemical level that can't be expressed or burnt through in other ways.

This becomes problematic when systems like our justice system don't recognise that these behaviours are a response to living with the results of trauma. In young people it's classified as destructive behaviour, which leads them straight into the juvenile justice system. We have too many Aboriginal and Torres Strait Islander children getting locked up for trauma-fuelled behaviours.

'Lateral violence' often arises from a feeling of scarcity. If you are a minority group, or you've experienced scarcity due to structural racism or government policy, you may find there is a lot of competition for limited resources such as employment or funding for projects and this can lead to lateral violence. The original work that identified lateral or horizontal violence was done in a nursing context (Duffy, 1995; Griffin, 2004). It is defined as 'overt and covert non-physical hostility such as sabotage, infighting, scapegoating and criticism' (Duffy, 1995, p. 5). Duffy's premise was to see nurses structurally as an oppressed group, which makes the term 'lateral violence' relevant for First Nations people who have long suffered the oppression of colonisation (see Clark et al., 2016; Clark & Glover, 2019; Whyman et al., 2021).

The following story of the Great Murray Cod, told to Nicole as part of her Honours thesis, is how Gamilaroi man Clinton Schultz explains lateral violence in Aboriginal communities:

> For me [lateral violence] is like what I've been witnessing in our waterways... down on our Country between the Great Murray Cod and the Carp. That cod, he swam around forever, he didn't have too many worries, he was protective of his areas but didn't go out of his way to attack his own, just maintained ... protection of his own little river or the dam or the lake. He was an apex predator without many concerns. Then all of a sudden, someone came along and dropped a carp in that river. And carps are damn good survivors as well and an apex predator from somewhere else. The carp survived in a different way but, instead of just maintaining his own little patch...his method of survival was to eat as much as possible and multiply as quick as possible. He just started chewing up other parts of the river, spreading further and further, getting bigger and bigger, and slowly but surely that Murray Cod had to back up into further little corners. He'd be watching that carp and just seeing how he was surviving and getting to that stage that there were such limited resources left for him, that he started to believe that "if I'm gonna survive, I've gotta live like that carp". And all of sudden, they started eating their own, something they'd never been doing. The Murray Cod start turning around and eating their own, their young ones, out of that fear of not surviving, not having enough resource. So essentially, what ended up happening [was that] while that Cod's maintained his shape, maintained his form, he's actually forgotten what it means to be a cod. He's just become that carp. It's not that he's bad [or] because he's evil, he's just learned that's what he has to do to survive. Unfortunately. (Cited in Tujague, 2018, p. 66).

## Polyvagal Theory and the Vagus Nerve

As First Nations Peoples, we know that our traditional practices such as dancing, singing, drumming and meditation are powerful and nurturing. Embedded deep within these elements of culture is the nurturing of the vagus nerve whose two branches travel through the head, neck, chest, and abdomen (highlighted in yellow in Fig. 4.6), listening and talking to the heart, lungs and stomach. It plays an essential role in how we perceive and relate to one another and how we respond to threat. The vagus nerve, so vital to our health and existence, can be massaged from the inside through activities such as our traditional practices.

Dr Stephen Porges' 'polyvagal theory' (Porges, 2001, 2011), takes us deeper into what we now understand about the nervous system and our

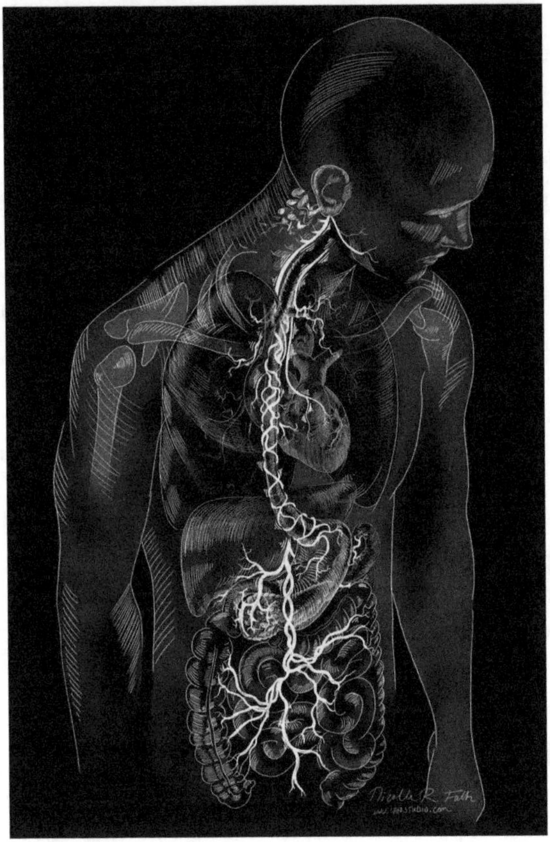

**Fig. 4.6** The vagus nerve

evolution as social beings. Polyvagal theory helps to explain the function and impact of the vagus nerve on our social interaction and threat response. Recall that we talked earlier in the chapter about the body in terms of its central nervous system and its autonomic nervous system and went further in dividing the autonomic nervous system into two complementary nervous systems, the sympathetic (arousing) and parasympathetic (calming) nervous systems.

The parasympathetic nervous system houses both branches of the vagus nerve, the dorsal (back) complex, and the ventral (front) complex.

The ventral complex is newer than the dorsal complex; it is protected by a myelin sheath which allows messages to travel faster along it. It innervates many parts of the body above the diaphragm that help us to connect to others, for example, its web of nerve fibres enables our voice, hearing and facial expressions.

According to polyvagal theory, because we are social beings, we always go first to befriend and if that doesn't work, we move through fight or flight and then freeze or shut down. The length of time we will invest in befriending can be short, ending after only seconds at the quick recognition of a snarl on another's lips or an ingenuine glint in their eye. On the other hand, it may form our long-term strategy for survival.

The dorsal complex, the older branch of the vagus nerve, innervates organs below the diaphragm including the gut. Eighty percent of the vagus nerve fibres take information from the body to the brain, with only twenty percent of the fibres taking information from the brain to the body. This perhaps explains why new research refers to the gut as 'the second brain' (Mayer, 2011). It also makes us appreciate the importance of trusting our 'gut feelings', something that modern society does not give a lot of credit to.

## Polyvagal Theory and the Threat Response

Polyvagal theory supports the theory that we go through a hierarchy of three stages when we are confronted with threat. At the top of the hierarchy, we operate in the ventral complex where we feel safe and socially connected. When the ventral complex of the vagus nerve is active, we look for social contact which activates the parasympathetic nervous system, bringing us towards balance and calm. This is when we are in 'befriend', the first response of our nervous system to keep us safe.

When finding safety in social connections doesn't work, our sympathetic nervous system floods our body with hormones to mobilise us for fight or flight. It is the dorsal complex, the most primal branch of the vagus nerve whose fibres reach into our hearts, lungs and stomach, that steps in and becomes active. The sympathetic system is aroused and continues to build unless the threat resolves. If the threat is not resolved the sympathetic arousal can become so extreme that the body is unable to cope. At this point, the fail-safe survival mechanism kicks in. While the dorsal complex normally serves to gently modulate between arousal and relaxation, when the sympathetic system is too aroused, the dorsal complex spikes and overwhelms the sympathetic system, shutting the system down, sending the person into what we commonly call 'freeze'.

Another type of threat response you may have heard of is 'fawn'. This term was first coined by Pete Walker (2013). Someone who goes to fawn to survive, befriends the perpetrator to the extent that they are submissively co-dependent. This may mean they sacrifice self-identity and healthy personal boundaries, appeasing the perpetrator to avoid rejection.

The tone of the vagus nerve influences the tone of every organ it innervates. Humming is one activity that is great for massaging and stimulating the vagus nerve. Others are gargling and singing at the top of your voice.

**Activity 4.2 Humming**

When you're humming, what you're looking for is vibration in your lips and mouth and throat. We know that deep humming, that deep chanting hum that monks do, is the *only* thing that massages your heart, the hardest working muscle in your body (Nikhil Kumar et al., 2018). A lot of cultures use humming. When people do yoga, they use the 'om' as a type of hum.

Take some time to hum now... do it for about one or two minutes. Take deep breaths in and hum as you let each breath out. Deep breathing balances the autonomic nervous system. One of the techniques we use with kids who are really upset or hyper-aroused is to get them to go outside and blow bubbles or hum or even whistle. Those activities get them breathing in and breathing out more deeply, instead of that shallow breathing that happens when they are hyper-aroused. These are all examples of sensory-motor exercises.

**Activity 4.3 Trauma and the Brain**

This is a great video clip (Fig. 4.7) that sums up everything we talk about in this chapter. Think about these three questions while you're watching the clip:

- How did the traumatic event affect the young woman's memory?
- Which part of the brain was calculating if there was time for another drink before the next train?
- What was one grounding technique they suggest in the video clip?

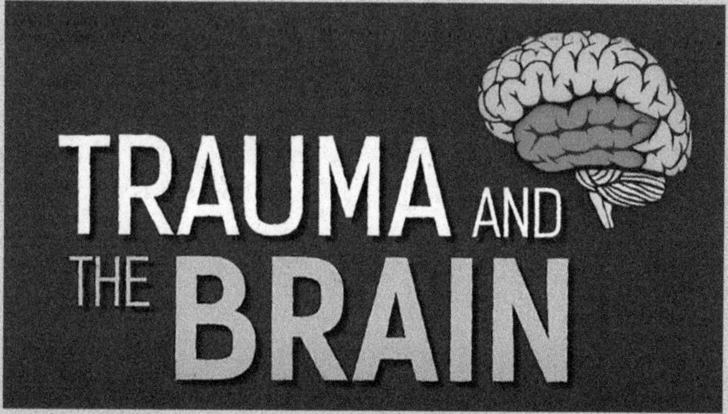


Fig. 4.7 Trauma and the Brain video – Produced by media co-op and NHS Lanarkshire. Source: https://www.youtube.com/watch?v=4-tcKYx24aA

***Nicole:*** *The part of the video I always reflect on is when the police officers went back after their trauma training and asked the young woman, "What can you remember? Tell us anything you can remember?" and she says, "Cigarette smoke, I can smell it now." And I know from our work with trauma survivors that so many people talk about smell and how what they could smell at the time of the trauma event triggers their memory of that event.*

***Kelleigh****: What I love about the clip is the job they've done in bringing all the parts together. We know that you don't make memories in a linear fashion when you're in fight, flight or freeze, but you do make them depending on the emotional content, the emotional arousal or threat to the person.*

That's problematic in our legal system where the victim of a rape, say, would traditionally be asked, "What happened next? And what happened after that? Why didn't you fight back?" When we've done this training with lawyers, they start to recognise that trauma memory is not linear. Now the legal profession as a whole is starting to incorporate what we know about trauma, understanding that you may not remember everything in a linear fashion, and that you may have been in hypo-arousal or freeze, which explains *why* you didn't run away or fight back.

## The Impact of Early Traumatic Experiences

We know that how your body responds depends on what resources you have emotionally, physically and socially. These resources will influence how well you recover and how quickly you heal from trauma. What happens to you in your early years impacts the resources that you have available to you. This is why at the close of this chapter we introduce you to the evidence from studies that link poor physical health to traumatic experiences in childhood and move from there to our understandings of the important role that attachment plays in psychological health. These studies and concepts form the basis of developmental trauma, which we discuss at the next billabong.

## The ACE Study

The ACE Study, published in 1998 (Felitti et al., 1998), describes research into how Adverse Childhood Experiences (ACEs) affect health across a lifetime. The implications of this research are well explained in a TED talk with Dr Nadine Burke Harris (Fig. 4.8), a paediatrician who works with young children in California. When we first saw this TED talk and learned about the ACE Study, we realised how important these insights are for our work in cultural safety in trauma-informed practice.

We ask you to take some time out now to watch this TED talk. If this information is new to you, we suggest you watch it with someone else, especially if you are Indigenous or have a trauma background. If you want to share it with friends and family, don't just send them the link without talking it through with them first; prepare them, make sure they watch it with someone; call them afterwards.

**Activity 4.4 Reflections on the Video**

Now think and reflect on these questions with someone:

- Did any of this information particularly shock you?
- What does knowing this information mean for you, your family and your community?

**Fig. 4.8** How childhood trauma affects health across the lifetime TED talk by Nadine Burke Harris (https://youtu.be/95ovIJ3dsNk)

***Kelleigh***: *I came across the ACE study years ago and it was one of those points in time where it made shocking sense. It validated a lot of what people knew anecdotally but had never had non-Indigenous science to back it up. It gave legitimacy to a lot of what we knew about intergenerational trauma and chronic illness that up until the results from the study were published, was really all about deficit and victim blaming. When I first watched this TED talk, I became quite distressed and had to leave the room. I was full of anger and sadness. I just kept thinking, "how long have we known this and we still do what we do to people?"*

*Another thing that struck me was that the study focused more on the links between childhood trauma and physiological health issues like heart disease and cancer, than on mental health. But if it wasn't for this study, we wouldn't know half of what we know now about treating trauma. We wouldn't have the treatment plans we have now. It would have taken forever for all of the different disciplines to come together, like medicine, social work, speech pathology and occupational therapy. The results of this study have forced us all to come together and have a collective approach in multidisciplinary teams.*

***Nicole***: *For me, the first thing I thought was: "this is why the gap won't close in the health disparities between Indigenous and non-Indigenous* *people". It seems so obvious and yet it seems difficult to incorporate into our policy making. I also felt relief, because if everyone understands what drives addictive behaviours, it should make it much easier to remove that stigma and work with it.*

We have had different reactions from people when we show this video in our face-to-face training. Some are concerned about labelling people, while others think it makes sense of what they see in their practice rooms and communities. For many people, this knowledge is life-changing: "oh my God, that's me, that's my life, that explains a lot".

## Attachment Theory

From the ACE study and others like it, we get a picture of how traumatic early childhood events impact on the *physical* resources you have available to you to live out a healthy life. Attachment Theory, which came out of experiments with monkeys done in the late 1950s, shows us how what happens to us in early childhood impacts on the emotional, social and psychological resources we have available to help us heal. John Bowlby (1988), one of the first people to develop the main concepts in Attachment Theory, was influenced by the study of animal family behaviours and later animal experiments done by Harry Harlow and Robert Zimmermann (1959). This was a time when people generally thought that what happened to children didn't influence their development into adulthood. Kids were thought to be pretty much a blank slate: you taught them what they needed to know and as long as they were fed and sheltered, they would be fine. Government policies in the past legitimised these ideas, built on the 'science' that as long as you feed your child and clothe and house them, they would be fine. However, when Harlow and Zimmermann did experiments with orphaned rhesus monkeys, what they found was something very different (Fig. 4.9).

What Harlow and Zimmermann did was create two pretend mummy monkeys and separate them from other monkeys. One was covered in soft, furry towelling and the other one was covered in just a wire shell. The monkey with the wire body had a bottle, so the little monkeys could get sustenance. The other one had a furry cover, which gave comfort, but

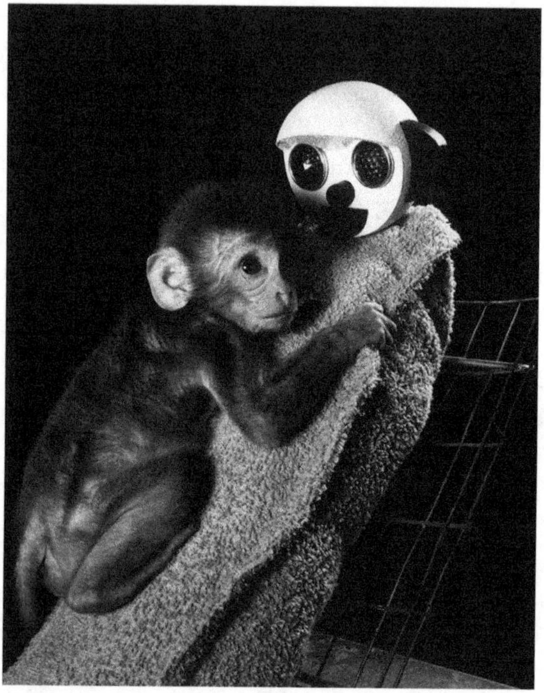

**Fig. 4.9** Rhesus monkey with cloth mother

no sustenance. The researchers assumed they would see the baby monkeys go to the mummy monkey which had food, because of course they would choose food over connection. But that's not what happened. The poor little monkeys would, out of desperation, drink from the wire monkey, but rush back to the other soft monkey for comfort and tactile connection.

Unfortunately, these little monkeys had ongoing changes to their behaviours. Some did not interact with the others again and some died refusing to eat and even self-mutilated (Zhang, 2017). While those experiments were extremely cruel and unethical, they changed the way we thought about childhood development and human interaction. Harlow (1958) in particular was interested in the 'nature of love' and was the first mainstream psychologist to make the claim that "the initial love responses of the human being are those made by the infant to the mother or some mother surrogate" (p. 673).

It's important to remember that the beliefs, that children only needed to be clothed and fed, were predominant in Australian society at the time of these experiments. Those beliefs would have led to broad unquestioning acceptance of the policy of forced removal of Aboriginal and Torres Strait Islander children from their families, which began in the mid 1800s and continued through to the 1970s. Later, non-Indigenous science realised something that collective communities have always known: well-being is *all* about attachment. It's *all* about safety, connection, comfort and relationship.

What we also know, years later, is that when you're born, your brain is just this mass of developing neurons waiting to form neural networks (Stiles & Jernigan, 2010). If you don't get interaction with your caregiver, if you don't get any response, if you don't get love, if you don't get connection, you don't grow the same type of neural networks as children who have all of those experiences. This means the whole foundation of your brain's neural network develops differently without this early connection to safety, comfort, mirroring and love.

## Attachment Styles

Your early childhood experiences influence how you feel about *you* in the world: are you worthy or unworthy? Is the world a safe or unsafe place? These experiences influence what your attachment 'style' will be (Bartholomew & Horowitz, 1991). Once you understand your attachment *style*, you get to understand why you chose that first partner, or why you might keep choosing the same type of partner. Once you understand your own attachment style, you can start to make different choices about relationships. Attachment styles experienced in adulthood will depend on what type of attachment developed in childhood.

Psychologists have identified two main types of attachment developed in early childhood: 'secure' and 'insecure' attachment. **Secure attachment** happens when the caregiver responds to the baby's cries in a consistent, safe and caring way. That child grows, knowing that if mum or dad or their caregiver disappear out of sight, they will come back. Their core belief becomes: *the world is a safe place*. **Insecure attachment** develops from when the child cries and no one attends, either because their caregiver chooses *not* to attend or they are *unable* to attend, that child comes to feel the world is *not* a safe place: "*you can cry out but no one's going to come, so why bother*?"

Adults with a 'secure' attachment style, can usually form loving and trusting relationships with others, while having little fear of being alone. While there is only one type of secure attachment style, psychologists have identified three main types of insecure attachment styles (with slightly different names) that feature in adult relationships (Bartholomew & Horowitz, 1991):

- **anxious attachment**, based on a deep fear of abandonment, fearing their partner will leave, always needing reassurance and validation (also called *anxious-ambivalent* or *anxious-preoccupied* attachment styles)
- **avoidant attachment**, based on a fear of closeness and intimacy, having difficulty getting close or trusting others (also called *dismissive-avoidant* or *anxious-avoidant* attachment styles)
- **fearful-avoidant attachment**, a combination of anxious and avoidant styles, simultaneously craving affection and wanting to avoid it (also called *disorganised attachment*).

Disorganised or fearful-avoidant attachment is the attachment style most associated with the trauma of child removal as a result of colonisation (Choate, et al., 2020). It is the most difficult to heal. This develops when sometimes the baby gets a good response and other times a harmful response from the caregiver. The child starts to learn that "if I cry, my caregiver might come, but they may not be safe and unless I'm really desperate, calling out is not a safe thing to do".

Even though attachment theory grew out of non-Indigenous psychology, understanding this notion of attachment styles is hugely important for our mob. How you formed your attachment early can influence everything you do throughout your life: what jobs you choose; what partners you take; how you live your life; what friendships you make; how you experience anxiety and depression. All are influenced by your attachment style, because they are critical to the foundations of your neural networks, the foundation of your brain and nervous system.

## Attachment in Individualist Cultures Vs. Collective Cultures

It's important to remember here that these understandings came about in a non-Indigenous, individualist-focused culture. What does that mean for us as First Nations Peoples of Australia? Think about the ongoing effects of colonisation in our country and what that means for *us*, because we are the children, grandchildren and great grandchildren of those young children who were taken away from their families and community caregivers. It's important to remember that, if we had been able to grow immersed in our culture, we would have been able to grow our neural networks like our ancestors, and things would be different today. This has also been the story for other First Nations Peoples who have experienced colonisation.

Aboriginal and Torres Strait Islander cultures, like all collective cultures, don't have attachment theories that mimic non-Indigenous attachment theories (Yeo, 2003). We have traditionally lived in collective groups and thrived under collective parenting and multiple caregivers—our aunties, our nannas, our siblings, our community. We have knowledge-holder roles, lore and ceremony that provide a symbiotic relationship environment of connection to all things. In Australia, like many other countries ruled by non-Indigenous policies, we have a child protection system that doesn't use our Indigenous attachment model (Yeo, 2003). It uses bits of it, like kinship care (Kiraly et al., 2015), but the main model and the main system works from the assumptions based on Bowlby's attachment theory.

If you are worried about the negative impacts of being taken from a caregiver and what that means, also think about what it means for our kids when we *do* have them in our families and at our gatherings. What's *that* doing to their brains, how's *that* growing them? Because our brains also have 'neural plasticity' or 'neuroplasticity' (Cozolino, 2014, 2017), they can grow new neural networks. We can grow those networks ourselves through the way we care for our kids and each other, through teaching our kids things, showing them love, encouraging them to learn themselves. We also know that if your brain has been damaged through a brain injury or trauma, you can train your brain to track around the damaged part (Evans & Coccoma, 2014).

Before colonisation, Aboriginal and Torres Strait Islander kids would have been taught to understand things like: 'where's the wind coming from; what's in season; where's the bird flying from; where are the bees heading to?' Those things would have formed a foundation of a neurological network that gave children a better understanding of spatial proximity. In the kinship system, each person involved in raising the child has their own roles. For example, the aunties might be responsible for teaching about relationships, or the eldest boy who goes through the coming-of-age ceremony may take more responsibility for younger children.

The box below adds more discussion from the literature on the differences between Indigenous and non-Indigenous understandings of attachment.

**Want to know more about attachment theory in individualist and collective cultures?**

Almost everyone who learns about attachment theory gets a bit freaked out. 'Oh, that's what I do with my kids'. 'Oh, that explains what happened to me. It can be useful to explain a lot of things about our own parenting and upbringing, but we must remember too, that a lot of these ideas and concepts are based in non-Indigenous values and understandings of the world. Research from Australia, New Zealand and Canada has shown that a lot of the underlying cultural assumptions of attachment theory don't always apply to the ways Indigenous peoples raise their kids. And yet these values continue to be used as the basis for decisions to remove Indigenous kids from their families and communities...

**Where did these ideas come from?**

It's good to get a sense of the context in which these ideas and theories developed. They were pretty radical when they first appeared in the 1950s. **John Bowlby** (1988) was the first to come up with theories based on the importance of a 'warm, intimate and continuous relationship' between a child and its mother (or 'permanent mother substitute') for the healthy psychological development of the child. Interestingly, Bowlby was born to upper class English parents in 1907 and had that warm relationship with a nanny, rather than his mother, like so many upper-class English kids. He was also sent to boarding school at the age of 7, a practice still common in that class of English society. When his much-loved nanny left the family when he was four, Bowlby described this 'as tragic as the loss of a mother' (Van Dijken, 1988, as cited in Wikipedia). Perhaps this is why he mentions the 'permanent mother substitute', which had not been the focus in earlier theories of child development.

(*continued*)

**(continued)**

Bowlby made his first formal statement of attachment theory in the first of three classic papers, titled *The Nature of the Child's Tie to his Mother* in 1958. Bowlby did not see attachment as a sign of dependency, as some theories of the time suggested, but rather that attachment performs a natural and healthy function, even into adulthood (Bretherton, 1992).

He followed this up with *Separation Anxiety*, published in 1959, drawing on detailed observations of children who had been separated from their parents through being in hospitals or institutions, as well as the results of those experiments with rhesus monkeys (Harlow & Zimmermann, 1959). He claimed that traditional theory could not explain the intense attachment young kids have with their mums nor their dramatic responses to being separated from them.

The third paper in the series, *Grief and Mourning in Infancy and Childhood*, published in 1960, caused the biggest stir. It challenged the theories of psychoanalysts like Anna Freud who believed that young kids who lose a parent 'cannot mourn because of insufficient ego development' (Bretherton, 1992, p. 763). Bowlby argued instead that mourning in infants occurs when they experience separation and the 'attachment figure', like the mum, continues to be unavailable.

Another important contribution to attachment theory was made by **Mary Ainsworth**, a Canadian researcher who joined Bowlby's research team in London in 1950. She developed the concept of the attachment figure as a secure base from which infants can explore the world (Bretherton, 1992). A very meticulous observer, she was also the initiator of the idea that the mum's sensitivity to her baby's signals is significant in the patterns of attachment that develop between mums and their babies. She is also recognised as the first to come up with the four types of attachment style still used today: secure, avoidant, fearful-avoidant and anxious.

**Different cultures, different values**

While there is no doubt that all babies, no matter what culture they are born into, seek out closeness with their caregivers for protection and care, how those caregivers give that protection depends on the values of the cultures in which that care takes place. One of the most influential papers that raised questions about the so-called 'universality' of attachment theory across cultures was published in 2000 by American and Japanese psychologists, who called for 'an indigenous approach to the psychology of attachment' (Rothbaum et al., 2000, p. 1093).

A study by psychologist Soo See Yeo (2003) is one of the first to explore how appropriate it is to use attachment theory as a basis for removing Australian Aboriginal kids. Yeo yarned with Aboriginal people about the practicalities of raising kids in both urban areas and the bush. From these yarns, Yeo came up with ways that mainstream and Aboriginal values around child rearing are different.

(*continued*)

**(continued)**

**Values underpinning the three core hypotheses of attachment theory**

Criticisms about how relevant attachment theory is to the way Indigenous families and communities raise their kids centre around the difference in values that lie behind what psychologists call the 'three core hypotheses' (Rothbaum et al., 2000): the sensitivity hypothesis, the competence hypothesis and the secure base hypothesis. Yeo's study uses the Rothbaum critique of the three core hypotheses as a framework to explain the differences between mainstream and Aboriginal values.

**Sensitivity hypothesis**

Attachment theory says that babies and young children become securely or insecurely attached depending mainly on the mother's ability to sensitively respond to the signals the baby gives, like crying. That means mum waits for bub to cry before she does anything. What Mary Ainsworth described as sensitive, responsive caregiving reflects the non-Indigenous value placed on children's autonomy and self-expression (Rothbaum et al., 2000). In Aboriginal and Torres Strait Islander cultures, where there are often many carers (aunties and uncles, grandparents, brothers and sisters), sensitivity means anticipating their babies' needs, making sure they are comfortable and their needs are met, before they need to cry (Yeo, 2003). Non-Indigenous values may interpret this anticipation as indulging or 'spoiling' the kids, preventing them from developing their independence.

**Competence hypothesis**

Attachment theory says that if kids are secure, they will grow up to be more socially and emotionally competent than kids who didn't grow up with secure attachments. Competence means things like being independent, able to regulate emotions and able to express themselves. Rather than valuing competence in terms of independence and self-expression, Yeo's Aboriginal participants talked about the importance of interdependence, group cohesion and loyalty, spiritual connectedness, traditional links to country and inter-assistance (family and community responsibilities for kids) as indicators of social and emotional competence.

**Secure base hypothesis**

Attachment theory says that a child will explore their environment and develop independence when they have a 'secure base' provided by the protective presence of their mum or caregiver. Yeo argues that security for an Aboriginal child is based on a network of regular caregivers, which 'allows the support and maintenance of the child's emotional health through their lifespan' (Yeo, 2003, p. 299). Studies such as those by Malin et al. (1996) and Priest et al. (2007) also found that Aboriginal children up to two years of age are discouraged from exploring, being carried rather than encouraged to crawl or walk. On the other hand, older brothers and sisters were encouraged to be self-reliant, while looking out for younger kids. According to Ryan (2011, p. 188), this 'suggests that peers and multiple caregivers may act as a secure base'.

(*continued*)

**(continued)**

**What does this mean for our mob?**

The implications of these cultural differences are particularly important when it comes to making 'assessments' based on mainstream notions of attachment and bonding that then lead to decisions about removing children from their parents and communities. Yeo's findings are supported by research in Indigenous cultures in Canada and New Zealand as well as Australia (see reference list at the end of the chapter). What is common to Indigenous cultures is that attachment occurs in a collective cultural context, which includes connection to ancestors, land and spirit. Children are rarely raised by one or two caregivers, as is assumed in the nuclear family-centric notions that underpinned the theories and research undertaken by Bowlby and Ainsworth. Littlebear (2000) describes this kinship as a 'spider web of relations' (cited in Carriere & Richardson, 2009, p.55), a kinship that extends beyond human relationships to connection with the natural world, where social obligations involve 'reciprocity in relationship with plants and animals' (Carriere & Richardson, 2009, p. 55).

**Activity 4.5 Reflective Questions on Attachment Theory**

- What ideas from Attachment Theory make the most sense to you?
- What ideas about raising healthy kids were present in your family and community when you grew up?
- How much does Attachment Theory help explain your own experiences as a child and a parent?
- How could you use your understanding of Attachment Theory in your work?

## Concluding Comments

At this billabong we have dived deep into some of the most important information we need to understand trauma, including: its impact on the brain and the entire body system; how the body responds when there is danger or a threat; and how those responses can become habitual and ingrained. The most far-reaching impact of trauma results from trauma in early childhood. We looked at the ACE Study, and Attachment Theory to get a clearer picture of how this plays out in later life. For First Nations Peoples the impact of the forced removals of children have created mass collective trauma. In the next chapter we cover in more detail the different types of trauma that affect First Nations Peoples as a direct result of colonisation. But first, take a moment to do the following simple and calming grounding exercise:

**Activity 4.6 Swaying**

If you're sitting down, stand up. Place your feet apart just under your hips and bend your knees a little. Now move your weight from side to side. Don't hurt yourself. Just sway nice and gently.

This can be very good for calming your system and getting rid of some the nervous energy from your body. This is a sensory-motor grounding exercise.

**Activity 4.7 Check out and Reflection**

Check in with your body and think about how you're feeling and where you feel it. Then write some answers to these reflective questions:

- What was the main thing that challenged your knowledge system in this chapter?
- How did your knowledge system grow from learning this information?
- How will you use the knowledge you've taken from this billabong?
- What difference could this knowledge make to your family and community life?

## References and Further Reading

American Psychiatric Association. (2013). *Diagnostic and statistical manual of mental disorders* (5th ed.).

Atkinson, S., & Swain, S. (1999). A network of support: Mothering across the Koorie community in Victoria, Australia. *Women's History Review, 8*(2), 219–230.

Bartholomew, K., & Horowitz, L. M. (1991). Attachment styles among young adults: A test of a four-category model. *Journal of Personality and Social Psychology, 61*(2), 226–244. https://doi.org/10.1037/0022-3514.61.2.226

Bessarab, D., & Crawford, F. (2010). Aboriginal practitioners speak out: Contextualising child protection interventions. *Australian Social Work, 63*(2), 179–193.

Bowlby, J. (1988). *A secure base: Parent-child attachment and healthy human development*. Basic Books.
Bremner, J. D. (2006). Traumatic stress: Effects on the brain. *Dialogues in Clinical Neuroscience, 8*(4), 445. https://doi.org/10.31887/DCNS.2006.8.4/jbremner
Bretherton, I. (1992). The origins of attachment theory: John Bowlby and Mary Ainsworth. *Developmental Psychology, 28*(5), 759–775.
Buchheim, A., George, C., Gündel, H., & Viviani, R. (2017). Neuroscience of human attachment. *Frontiers in Human Neuroscience, 11*, 1–136. https://doi.org/10.3389/fnhum.2017.00136
Cannon, W. B. (1914). The emergency function of the adrenal medulla in pain and the major emotions. *American Journal of Physiology-Legacy Content, 33*(2), 356–372.
Carriere, J., & Richardson, C. (2009). From longing to belonging: Attachment theory, connectedness, and Indigenous children in Canada. In S. Mckay, D. Fuchs, & I. Brown (Eds.), *Passion for action in child and family services: Voices from the Prairies* (pp. 49–67). Canadian Plains Research Centre.
Carrión, V. G., Haas, B. W., Garrett, A., Song, S., & Reiss, A. L. (2010). Reduced hippocampal activity in youth with posttraumatic stress symptoms: An fMRI study. *Journal of Pediatric Psychology, 35*(5), 559–569. https://doi.org/10.1093/jpepsy/jsp112
Choate, P. W., Kohler, T., Cloete, F., CrazyBull, B., Lindstrom, D., & Tatoulis, P. (2019). Rethinking *Racine v Woods* from a decolonizing perspective: Challenging the applicability of attachment theory to Indigenous families involved with child protection. *Canadian Journal of Law and Society/Revue Canadienne Droit et Société, 34*(1), 55–78.
Choate, P. W., CrazyBull, B., Lindstrom, D., & Lindstrom, G. (2020). Where do we go from here?: Ongoing colonialism from Attachment Theory. *Aotearoa New Zealand Social Work, 32*(1), 32–44.
Clark, Y., & Glover, K. (2019). Lateral violence in Aboriginal communities: From awareness to transformations. In Y. Clark & K. Glover (Eds.), *Harnessing the transformative power of education* (pp. 16–35). Brill Sense.
Clark, Y., Augoustinos, M., & Malin, M. (2016). Lateral violence within the Aboriginal community in Adelaide: "It affects our identity and wellbeing". *Journal of Indigenous Wellbeing, 1*(1), 43–52.
Cozolino, L. (2014). *The neuroscience of human relationships: Attachment and the developing social brain*. WW Norton & Company.
Cozolino, L. (2017). *The neuroscience of psychotherapy: Healing the social brain* (3rd ed.). WW Norton & Company.

Donoghue, E. (2010). *Room*. HarperCollins.

Duffy, E. (1995). Horizontal violence: A conundrum for nursing. *Collegian, 2*(2), 5–17. https://doi.org/10.1016/S1322-7696(08)60093-1

Eriksson, M., Ghazinour, M., & Hammarström, A. (2018). Different uses of Bronfenbrenner's ecological theory in public mental health research: What is their value for guiding public mental health policy and practice? *Social Theory & Health, 16*(4), 414–433.

Evans, A., & Coccoma, P. (2014). *Trauma-informed care: How neuroscience influences practice*. Routledge.

Fast, E., & Collin-Vézina, D. (2019). Historical trauma, race-based trauma, and resilience of indigenous peoples: A literature review. *First Peoples Child & Family Review, 14*(1), 166–181.

Felitti, V. J., Anda, R. F., Nordenberg, D., Williamson, D. F., Spitz, A. M., Edwards, V., & Marks, J. S. (1998). Relationship of childhood abuse and household dysfunction to many of the leading causes of death in adults: The Adverse Childhood Experiences (ACE) Study. *American Journal of Preventive Medicine, 14*(4), 245–258.

Fleming, A. (2016). *In what ways are indigenous Māori perspectives on attachment similar to and different from western psychoanalytic perspectives on attachment and what are the implications for the practice of psychotherapy in Aotearoa New Zealand?* (Master of Psychotherapy), Auckland University of Technology, Auckland.

Griffin, M. (2004). Teaching cognitive rehearsal as a shield for lateral violence. *Journal of Continuing Education in Nursing, 35*(6), 257–263.

Harlow, H. F. (1958). The nature of love. *American Psychologist, 13*(12), 673–685.

Harlow, H. F., & Zimmermann, R. R. (1959). Affectional responses in the infant monkey. *Science, 130*(3373), 421–432.

Herman, J. L. (2015). *Trauma and recovery: The aftermath of violence--from domestic abuse to political terror*. Hachette UK.

Jones, L. K., & Cureton, J. L. (2014). Trauma redefined in the DSM-5: Rationale and implications for counseling practice. *Professional Counselor, 4*(3), 257–271.

Ketheesan, S., Rinaudo, M., Berger, M., Wenitong, M., Juster, R. P., McEwen, B. S., & Sarnyai, Z. (2020). Stress, allostatic load and mental health in Indigenous Australians. *Stress, 23*(5), 509–518. https://doi.org/10.1080/10253890.2020.1732346

Kezelman, C., Hossack, N., Stavropoulos, P., & Burley, P. (2015). *The cost of unresolved childhood trauma and abuse in adults in Australia*. Adults Surviving Child Abuse and Pegasus Economics.

Kiraly, M., James, J., & Humphreys, C. (2015). 'It's a family responsibility': Family and cultural connection for Aboriginal children in kinship care. *Children Australia, 40*(1), 23–32. https://doi.org/10.1017/cha.2014.36

Levy, K. N., Hlay, J. K., Johnson, B. N., & Witmer, C. P. (2019). An attachment theoretical perspective on tend-and-befriend stress reactions. *Evolutionary Psychological Science, 5*(4), 426–439. https://doi.org/10.1007/s40806-019-00197-x

MacLean, P. D. (1990). *The triune brain in evolution: Role in paleo cerebral functions.* Plenum.

Maddi, S. R. (2002). The story of hardiness: Twenty years of theorizing, research, and practice. *Consulting Psychology Journal: Practice and Research, 54*(3), 173–185. https://doi.org/10.1037/1061-4087.54.3.173

Maier, S. F., & Seligman, M. E. (1976). Learned helplessness: Theory and evidence. *Journal of Experimental Psychology: General, 105*(1), 3–46.

Malin, M., Campbell, K., & Agius, L. (1996). Raising children in the Nunga Aboriginal way. *Family Matters, 43*, 43–47.

Mayer, E. A. (2011). Gut feelings: The emerging biology of gut–brain communication. *Nature Reviews Neuroscience, 12*(8), 453–466.

Neal, J. W., & Neal, Z. P. (2013). Nested or networked? Future directions for ecological systems theory. *Social Development, 22*(4), 722–737.

Nikhil Kumar, M., Koushik, K., & Deepak, K. (2018). Prediction of heart diseases using data mining and machine learning algorithms and tools. *International Journal of Scientific Research in Computer Science Engineering and Information Technology, 3*(3).

Nirupama, R., Rajaraman, B., & Yajurvedi, H. N. (2018). Stress and Glucose metabolism: A review. *Imaging Journal of Clinical Medical Sciences, 5*(1), 008–012. https://doi.org/10.17352/2455-8702.000037

O'Brien, M. (2010). Towards integration. In S. Brown & R. Lent (Eds.), *Handbook of Counseling Psychology* (3rd ed., pp. 173–192). John Wiley & Sons.

O'Neill, L., Guenette, F., & Kitchenham, A. (2010). 'Am I safe here and do you like me?' Understanding complex trauma and attachment disruption in the classroom. *British Journal of Special Education, 37*(4), 190–197.

Overmars, D. (2010). Diagnosis as a naming ceremony: Caution warranted in use of the DSM-IV with Canadian Aboriginal Peoples. *First Peoples Child & Family Review, 5*(1), 78–85. https://doi.org/10.7202/1069064ar

Pai, A., Suris, A. M., & North, C. S. (2017). Posttraumatic stress disorder in the DSM-5: Controversy, change, and conceptual considerations. *Behavioral Sciences, 7*(1), 1–7. https://doi.org/10.3390/bs7010007

Perry, B. D. (2006). Fear and learning: Trauma-related factors in the adult education process. *New Directions for Adult and Continuing Education, 2006*(110), 21–27. https://doi.org/10.1002/ace.215

Perry, B. D. (2008). Child maltreatment: A neurodevelopmental perspective on the role of trauma and neglect in psychpathology. In T. P. Beauchaine & S. P. Hinshaw (Eds.), *Child and Adolescent Psychopathology* (pp. 93–128). John Wiley & Sons Inc.

Perry, B. D. (2009). Examining child maltreatment through a neurodevelopmental lens: Clinical applications of the neurosequential model of therapeutics. *Journal of Loss and Trauma, 14*(4), 240–255. https://doi.org/10.1080/15325020903004350

Ploog, D. W. (2003). The place of the Triune Brain in psychiatry. *Physiology & Behavior, 79*(3), 487–493.

Porges, S. (2001). The polyvagal theory: Phylogenetic substrates of a social nervous system. *International Journal of Pyschophysiology, 42*(2), 123–146.

Porges, S. (2011). *The polyvagal theory: Neurophysiological foundations of emotions, attachment, communication and self-regulation.* Norton & Company.

Priest, K., King, S., Nungarrayi Brown, W., Nangala, I., & Nangala, M. (2007). Warrki Jarrinjaku Jintangkarmanu Purananjaku "Working together everyone and listening": Aboriginal child rearing in remote Central Australia. *Canadian Journal of Native Education, 30*, 61–74.

Roelofs, K. (2017). Freeze for action: Neurobiological mechanisms in animal and human freezing. *Philosophical Transactions of the Royal Society of London Series B, Biological Sciences, 372*(1718). https://doi.org/10.1098/rstb.2016.0206

Rothbaum, F., Weisz, J., Pott, M., Miyake, K., & Morelli, G. (2000). Attachment and culture: Security in the United States and Japan. *American Psychologist, 55*(10).

Ryan, F. (2011). Kanyininpa (Holding): A way of nurturing children in Aboriginal Australia. *Australian Social Work, 64*(2), 183–197.

Schoenemann, P. T. (2006). Evolution of the size and functional areas of the human brain. *Annual Review of Anthropology, 35*, 379–406.

Shapiro, R. (2010). *The trauma treatment handbook: Protocols across the spectrum.* WW Norton & Company.

Shapiro, R. (2020). *Doing psychotherapy: A trauma and attachment-informed approach.* WW Norton & Company.

Sheehan, N. (2012). *Stolen generations education: Aboriginal cultural strengths and social and emotional wellbeing.* Link-Up QLD.

Siegel, D. J. (1999). *The developing mind: Toward a neurobiology of interpersonal experience.* Guildford Press.

Siegel, D. J. (2012). *The developing mind: How relationships and the brain interact to shape who we are* (2nd ed.). Guildford Press.

Stiles, J., & Jernigan, T. L. (2010). The basics of brain development. *Neuropsychology Review, 20*(4), 327–348. https://doi.org/10.1007/s11065-010-9148-4

Sweeton, J. (2019). *The trauma treatment toolbox.* Pesi Publishing.

Taylor, S. E., Klein, L. C., Lewis, B. P., Gruenewald, T. L., Gurung, R. A. R., & Updegraff, J. A. (2000). Biobehavioral responses to stress in females: Tend-and-befriend, not fight-or-flight. *Psychological Review, 107*(3), 411–429.

Taylor, P., Moore, P., Pezzullo, L., Tucci, J., Goddard, C., & De Bortoli, L. (2008). *The cost of child abuse in Australia.* Melbourne: Australian Childhood Foundation and Child Abuse Prevention Research Australia.

Tronick, E. (2009). *Still face experiment: Dr Edward Tronick.* Retrieved from https://www.youtube.com/watch?v=apzXGEbZht0&feature=youtu.be

Tujague, N. (2018). *Why the gap won't close: Aboriginal and Torres Strait Islander consultants' perspectives on working at the cultural interface in community.* (Honours thesis), Southern Cross University, Lismore

Van der Kolk, B. A. (2015). *The body keeps the score: Brain, mind, and body in the healing of trauma.* Viking Press.

Van Dijken, S. (1988). *John Bowlby: His early life: A biographical journey into the roots of attachment theory.* Free Association Books.

Walker, P. (2013). *Complex PTSD: From surviving to thriving.* Azure Coyote.

Whyman, T., Adams, K., Carter, A., & Jobson, L. (2021). Lateral violence in Indigenous peoples. *Australian Psychologist, 56*(1), 1–14.

Yeo, S.-S. (2003). Bonding and attachment of Australian Aboriginal children. *Child Abuse Review, 12,* 292–304.

Yunkaporta, T., & Kirby, M. (2011). Yarning up Aboriginal pedagogies: A dialogue about eight Aboriginal ways of learning. In N. Purdie, G. Milgate, & H. R. Bell (Eds.), *Two way teaching and learning: Toward culturally reflective and relevant education* (pp. 205–213). ACER Press.

Yunkaporta, T., & McGinty, S. (2009). Reclaiming Aboriginal knowledge at the cultural interface. *The Australian Educational Researcher, 36*(2), 55–72. https://doi.org/10.1007/BF03216899

Zhang, B. (2017). Consequences of early adverse rearing experience (EARE) on development: Insights from non-human primate studies. *Zoological Research, 38*(1), 7–35.

# 5

# Sharing Trauma Knowledge: Types of Trauma

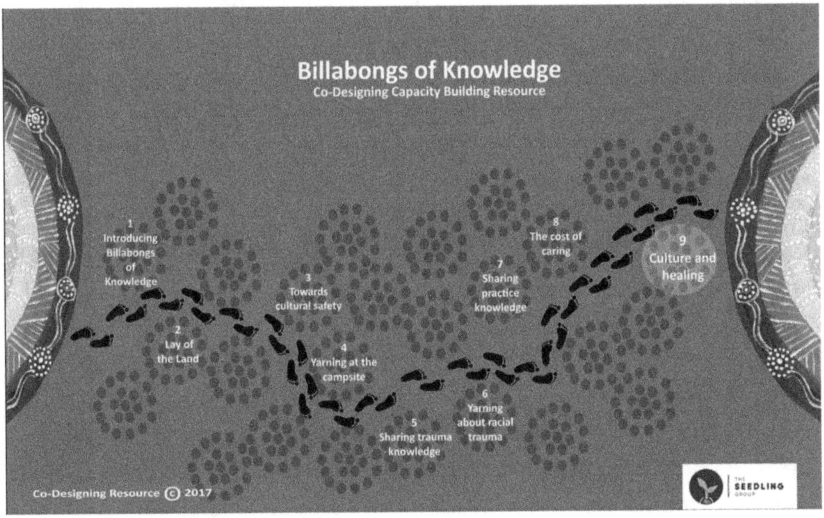


We acknowledge the traditional custodians of the land on which we work and live. We recognise their continuing connection to land, water, and community. We pay our respects to Elders past, present and emerging and extend that respect to all Aboriginal and Torres Strait Islander Peoples today.



N. Tujague, K. Ryan, *Cultural Safety in Trauma-Informed Practice from a First Nations Perspective*, https://doi.org/10.1007/978-3-031-13138-7_5

## Introduction

For First Nations Peoples across Australia, trauma began with the invasion of colonisation. We could say the first trauma was environmental trauma, encompassing all the other kinds of trauma we will talk about at this billabong. The intricate links between Country and Indigenous peoples were severely disrupted when lands were taken, fences put up, mines put down, waterholes and rivers poisoned, land degraded, people killed, children taken. From an Indigenous Knowledge perspective, the path to the crisis we all now face at the planetary level came from 'the direct appropriation of Indigenous peoples' ancestral lands' (Redvers et al., 2020, p. 2).

At the last billabong we set up camp and started to yarn about trauma. At this billabong we dig down into more detail and share knowledge around the different *types* of trauma people can experience. We distinguish 'single incident trauma', which can be relatively clear to understand, and which can build resilience, from the more complex types of trauma that First Nations Peoples have experienced as a direct result of colonisation. We explore developmental trauma that arises from the types of adverse childhood experiences we talked about in the previous chapter, especially child neglect.

We spend some time talking about the effect on the brain of PTSD (Post-Traumatic Stress Disorder) and explain how PTSD is a recurring response to the original trauma. We then go on to explore the different forms of complex trauma, including intergenerational, institutional, and collective trauma, all of which impact disproportionately on us as First Nations Peoples. We look into historical trauma in some depth and finish where we started this chapter, with a more detailed look at environmental trauma, the first trauma experienced by First Nations Peoples from the onset of colonisation.

**Activity 5.1 Check-in**

Remember the reason we check-in is to connect your mind and your body and be present. Take a minute to check in on how you are feeling, where you feel it in your body, and how you are showing up to this billabong. Simply honour how you're feeling in your body and in your mind.

**Activity 5.2 Stomping**

When you stomp it calms your nervous system. Stomping is a good exercise that moves your major muscle groups and uses up some of those hormones like adrenaline and cortisol in your body, but it also helps to engage the frontal lobes (neocortex) in problem-solving. Our mob have always been about moving and making noise through singing, connecting, dancing and other rituals. If you want to know more about moving major muscle groups and why that's helpful and important in grounding and dealing with trauma, have a look at the work of Bessel Van der Kolk (2014) and Peter Levine (2010).

One stomping exercise that's good to do in a group, is to have everyone stand in a circle and close their eyes. Then someone starts by stomping one leg and then the other, which would count as two stomps. The next person adds another stomp, which makes three. Keep going around the circle, each person adding one more stomp in turn. This is a great exercise to do with kids. It's a good way to get everyone calm in the classroom. It's also an example of a sensory-motor exercise.

## Why Categorise Trauma?

In the Western scientific tradition, we like to silo everything, giving each type of thing its own name and its own category. It's a way of making meaning in that system, to separate things from the whole. Categorising can be useful to help us understand what we're dealing with when we work with clients presenting with the effects of that big category 'trauma'. Some people talk about trauma in terms of 'little' trauma or 'big' trauma, but because everyone is different and copes in different ways, we look at trauma based on how it impacts on the individual within the collective. Therefore, we prefer to think of trauma as being on a continuum. In different Aboriginal and Torres Strait Islander groups in community we see overlapping layers of different types of trauma. Dissecting and defining the different types of trauma can be useful in the therapeutic relationship.

For First Nations Peoples, instead of the category, the whole comes first, and what was happening in the whole, in the collective, is what led to particular symptoms. Something is lost in the deconstructing. Collective, holistic views are bigger than the categories that make them up. What we know holistically is what makes us well. The sounds of the bird calls, the smells of seasonal flowers, all go into making you well. They tell you something about your connection to your environment, to the other living creatures. When we destroy the environment, you no longer hear those calls or smell those flowers, or eat those foods which your body is attuned to having.

If you come to me and you're feeling depressed and you're not sleeping, I can suggest you seek medications; I can offer exercises you can do before sleep; I can suggest aromatherapy. But this kind of help doesn't address the fact that you will never again have those sounds and smells in your environment that feed your being, that are part of your DNA and make you well. You will be forever dependent on different stimuli or multiple pseudo solutions. But if I were to take into account the bigger, holistic picture, I would say, where do you go to hear those sounds? Where do you go to smell those plants that feed your senses? It becomes about connecting you back to the environment that's good for you. This is about understanding the whole story of you and that healing from trauma is a whole of body and spirit recovery, not just a cognitive or behavioural change.

We now take a more detailed look at different types of trauma that are useful to unpack, especially as we move towards the more complex end of the spectrum.

## Single Incident Trauma

Trauma that is based on a single incident, such as a natural disaster (Fig. 5.1), doesn't necessarily change our view of the world as being a safe place. We might rationalise that it won't happen again. It's also something that is impersonal, meaning it's not something that happened between people. When you can rationalise why something bad has happened, it means that you've brought your frontal lobes back online; your thinking brain can make sense of it as an uncommon event and put it into your long-term memory. The thinking brain assesses the memory: "Okay, I know why that happened. This is not normal. It may not happen again. I can do this." Once it's been consigned to your long-term memory, it doesn't stay there to trigger you. Often single incident traumas stimulate resilience.

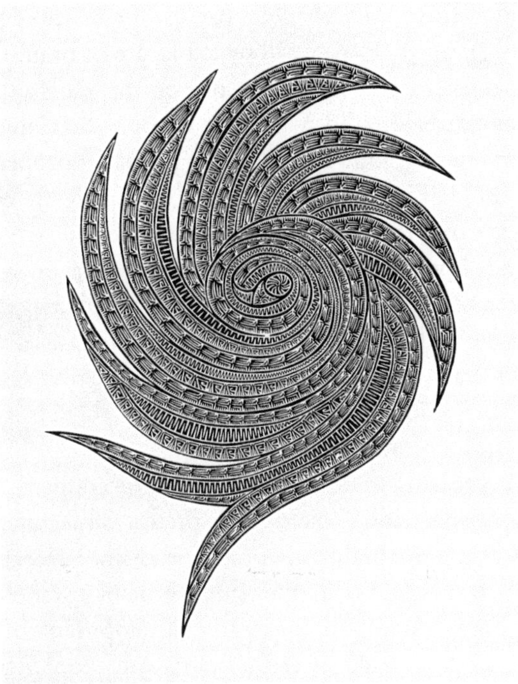

**Fig. 5.1** Marrkai Gub by Joel Sam with permission. The artists Impression of Cyclone Yasi

***Nicole**: We grew up in North Queensland where we had cyclones regularly. Kelleigh was just about to have her first baby when one of the cyclones hit. What we found was that when the next cyclone came, community really pulled together. People made sure everyone else had food. People made sure baths were full of water, windows were taped, all the usual things you do when there's a cyclone warning. The community-built resilience after that single incident trauma.*

## Developmental Trauma

We saw in the previous chapter the importance of understanding the impact of adverse childhood experiences on a child's development. This is at the core of developmental trauma, which happens during the time the child's brain is developing.

If you follow this link[1] to this paper on Bruce Perry's website (childtrauma.org), on p. 93 you will see a picture of brain images of two children, both at three years of age. The one on the left is a typical healthy brain of a three-year old child, while the one on the right is that of an orphan who suffered extreme neglect in an Eastern European orphanage (Perry, 2002, 2008; Beckett et al., 2006). The differences in size and structure indicate that there will also be differences in each child's ability and functioning. Looking more closely at these images, what we see is that the *institutionalised* child, the child from the orphanage, has a smaller brain, both in size and structure. This is an *extreme* case of neglect, when children's cries were rarely met with human contact (Beckett et al., 2006). Neglect of this magnitude provides evidence that there is a link between trauma, brain *structure* and brain *function*.

Some of the orphans in this story were later adopted and taken to homes that nourished and looked after them. While many did make some recovery and their brain functioning did improve, the brain sizes and functioning were always different from those of other children, influenced by the harm caused in that early development of their brains (Beckett et al., 2006). While healthy brains can usually find a way to work around structural damage from an injury or incident, brains that have experienced developmental trauma don't always have that capacity.

When one of the researchers visited that orphanage, he was struck by the silence (Weir, 2014). It felt so strange to hear no sounds in a place that housed young children. The researchers discovered what that really meant was the children had no reason to react or make a sound because when they did, no one came to help. This 'learned helplessness' (Maier & Seligman, 1976) has an obvious explanation: *there's no point in singing out if no one's going to come*. Another explanation is even more important: when the brain is developing, it's relying on all those neurons to make connections, but if there are no stimuli, the brain doesn't grow those connections.

A brain that isn't being used to learn or practise new things, either never develops those neural networks, or the under-utilised networks

[1] https://www.childtrauma.org/_files/ugd/aa51c7_471e37044892418589e6eb985bd2b027.pdf

shrink by a process called 'pruning' (Stamoulis et al., 2017). That's why neglect is so damaging. In those very early stages when the child's brain is developing, the more stimulus you give to that brain, the more little networks form, the better the brain growth and the healthier and more complex the whole system is. When your baby's born, and you say "hello!" and start talking to the child and laughing, making all those "goo goo" sounds, neural networks are being formed and the baby's learning things at an incredible speed. That developing brain is constantly relying on those stimuli and feedback loops to form its neural networks.

## The Body Remembers

We used to think that you couldn't remember things before the age of three or four. If you think back to your earliest memory, it was probably from around that age. Now we know that your brain and your body remember everything, but because you can't put words or a story to that memory, you can't recall it (Van der Kolk, 2014; Van der Kolk et al., 2009). Memories we can put stories to are called 'explicit' memories. They usually can be recalled after the age of two when verbal memory becomes established. Before you have language, you have 'implicit' memories or 'cellular' memories, so called because the body stores its memories in its cells. Cells change and store memories in a different way.

In the past, abusers have relied on the assumption that babies and very young children won't remember being abused. In fact, that young brain and that young body holds the memory in its cells and the trauma may play out later in life in different ways. Think back to the last billabong when we talked about befriend, fight, flight or freeze and what happens in the brain and the body. The cell remembers and encodes the trauma response, the memory in your limbic system, in your mid brain. It registers that the behaviour (of the abuser) brings pain. When retriggered, the adult or the child, who now has verbal abilities, may not be able to express or 'recall' what happened because they don't have a *verbal* memory even though they do have a *cellular* memory of that trauma event (Hartmann, 2019).

In hospitals we sometimes carry out invasive medical procedures on our children before and during birth. Within the first couple of minutes of life we jab them and prod them, which is all being registered by a developing brain that has never experienced this kind of pain before. A trauma history may present as hyperarousal or behavioural disorders. You might look at the family or the child's history, and think: "well, nothing's really happened that would make you think there's been trauma or that what we are seeing here is an expression of trauma". Trauma could have happened before, during, or after birth in that period before language is developed.

We need to ask ourselves exactly what's going on here. How much more careful and mindful should we be of the impact on that precious developing brain? A new-born baby immediately begins taking in their external environment and the stimuli from those around them. From the time of those early seconds, that child starts to know what's familiar and what's not familiar. If the face they see is responsible for hurting them, this will affect how their neural connections form. Even while that baby is growing in utero, everything that's taken into the baby's body is affecting not only the brain, but every organ of that developing baby. A lot of things can impact on the foetus, sometimes before a woman even knows she's pregnant (Buchheim et al., 2017).

## The Impact of Developmental Trauma on Language Development

Trauma, abuse and neglect affect language, another example of how trauma impacts on the developing brain (Allen & Oliver, 1982; Culp et al., 1991; Manso et al., 2010). Our sister Riley, who is a speech pathologist, tells us a story about a client she worked with, a young teenage girl who was finding it hard to both create friendship groups and keep her friends. The main issue that emerged was that the young person had a problem reading emotional cues. If a teenager has no idea about how to pick up emotional cues, she is likely to continue to find it hard to find and keep friends, which for a teenager is a big deal. There was trauma during early development leading to her inability to identify emotional cues with any consistency. She relied on her own reactions and she couldn't put herself in anyone else's shoes to imagine what they were thinking or feeling. For this teenager, she couldn't recognise peoples' changing emotions or an issue escalating from tone, expression or behaviour, so she was surprised when someone was suddenly angry. She had to rely on the literal meaning of the words people used when they spoke to her, which can be fraught in a teenage world. Once you recognise which skills haven't developed, it's possible to put in place a program that teaches the client skills and strategies. It can be hard work and it can be intricate, but it is possible to heal from trauma especially when you know at what developmental stage the trauma occurred.

It seems clear that the developmental stage at which the child experiences the trauma influences the skills they would normally be learning at that age. The difficulty is that the earlier in life that a child experiences trauma, the earlier the disruption to their expected development. If the trauma happens again and again, working out how to treat the original cause is complex, because it's very hard to find which part of that puzzle is missing. If developmental trauma is not identified at the time, children will often develop ways to work around what they may have missed. For this reason, the learning difficulty may only be picked up when the child has reached young adulthood.

What we've been learning in this section about developmental trauma can be very challenging, especially if you're in a parental or caregiving role. You may well be feeling regret or guilt. Remember, *we all do the best with the knowledge and resources we have available to us at the time.* It's important to recognise that because of the technology that allows us to see inside people's brains, we now have a much better understanding of what's going on when trauma happens, which means it's more possible now to create informed and positive interventions to reduce the impact of the damage.

**Activity 5.3 Clicking**

This might be a good moment to take some time out to re-balance yourself. Start with a few deep breaths. Now we will try to move some of that energy. First, think to yourself "you did the best you could with the knowledge and resources available to you at the time and you can heal from trauma." Next, we're going to click our fingers from left to right, right to left. Now, get a bit of a rhythm up. Let your body move, breathe in, breathe out, nice and slow. Keep doing that for as long as you're comfortable. Or you could go for a walk, make a cup of tea, grab some water, do whatever you need to do to calm your system.

When you're clicking, you're firstly shifting your focus between the left brain and right brain. You've also got some movement going on which activates those big muscle groups. You're activating your frontal lobes while you count and concentrate on the rhythm. You've got full activation, so you're burning through some of those chemicals, some of that stress hormone you've been releasing while you've been reading this. This is an example of a combination of a sensory-motor and cognitive grounding exercise.

## Post-traumatic Stress Disorder (PTSD)

The term PTSD (Post-Traumatic Stress Disorder), which almost everyone has heard of now, first appeared in the DSM in 1980 following research done with World War II and Vietnam war veterans. There is an interesting history to the idea that traumatic events, like disasters and wars, can create psychological problems. You might like to check out this history in a very readable paper written by psychiatrists Crocq and Crocq (2000). But it was in the first World War that terms like 'shell shock' (referring to exploding shells) were first used to explain symptoms like loss of memory and loss of vision following explosions. 'War neurosis' was another term used to describe experiences like recurring nightmares and flashbacks and emotional numbness. The importance of this resurfaced in World War II and later the Vietnam war, when symptoms of post-traumatic stress and re-traumatisation became so prevalent among war veterans.

For Aboriginal and Torres Strait Islander Peoples the experience is not unfamiliar. We hear people talk about being in 'deep pain'. Some traditional healers talk about people's spirits being out of alignment or having left them. We've heard this phenomenon described as people being 'ghosts walking their own land', they're here, but they're not here. While Western culture acknowledges all those lost in wars and the suffering from the impact of PTSD, there is little acknowledgement of the trauma resulting from the 'frontier wars' (Reynolds, 2013), fought by Australian Aboriginal Peoples in the first 140 years following colonisation.

## Triggering and Retriggering Explained

It's not uncommon to have some experience of retraumatising or retriggering from unresolved trauma. For example, someone might say something about you and you totally fly off the handle, becoming more reactive and emotional than that single comment warranted. Somehow, it touched something that happened to you before, which has triggered you to react in that way. In simple terms, retriggering or retraumatising means touching back on previous trauma. Even a trauma that's based in an implicit memory can retrigger you, which is why unearthing the source of the trigger can be so difficult.

To explain triggering in more detail, a trigger is a *sensory reminder of an unresolved traumatic event*. Triggers can be internal or external. An *internal trigger* can be a smell, a noise, the temperature, a taste, a touch, anything sensory that was present at the time of the traumatic event. An *external* trigger can be a place, an object, an argument, an ending of a relationship, too much to do, being overwhelmed, anniversaries, frightening news on the TV or even financial hardship.

These triggers can result in thoughts, feelings, or bodily sensations, like your heart racing, anything that's been encoded to that memory in your limbic system. Remember your limbic system never shuts down, as we talked about when we discussed the fear response in Chapter 4. While there may be gaps between limbic system information and memory, the connection is always there. When you experience a traumatic event, the memory is strongly encoded in the sensory stimuli so that it can be kept in your memory to keep you safe next time. Memory and stimulus are encoded together (Sotres-Bayon et al., 2006; Rogan et al., 1997).

When you haven't extinguished your fear response to a stimulus, you can, and will, continue to have a threat response whenever you encounter that stimulus, like Nicole and the fence. Even though it might be in a different context, the fear response, the memory and the stimulus are still encoded together. The association of the stimulus with the past trauma is still alive in your current response, *in the now*. When you see, or sense, the stimulus, your *whole body* has a threat response. This is *retriggering.*

Two things have to happen for you *not* to be retriggered by an external stimulus. The first one is the threat actually has to *stop*; you have to be safe. The second is you need to have your pre-frontal cortex, your thinking brain, online and available to you. This means you not only have the capacity to make sense of what's happened, but you are also able to take into account that you are in a different environment from the one where the traumatic event happened. You understand that while you're experiencing the same stimulus, you don't need to have the same response. Therefore, you can make sense of what's happening now and can extinguish, or at least reduce the activation (the way you react). You can feel safe in the *now* because your amygdala has given context to the stimulus (Evans & Coccoma, 2014).

A simple example: I see the spider, but I know it's plastic. If I'm looking at a plastic spider, I might still get that same fear response if I am scared of spiders, but I don't continue to act out and run away from it or try to kill it. This is an example of a response to a physical stimulus. You can however, have a panic attack by just thinking about the stimulus.

***Kelleigh:*** *I want to tell the story of a woman who talks to her amygdala when she feels a panic attack coming on. She says: "thank you for worrying about that for me; I get that you are looking out for me; but I'm here in my lounge room and I'm safe." Then she reaffirms context for her amygdala by breathing deeply and going through the five senses exercise. The more she does it, the easier it is for her to manage her threat response to that stimulus.*

## Trauma Brain Images

Since the arrival of brain imaging technology, we can see what is happening in the brain as a result of trauma and re-traumatisation. Figure 5.2

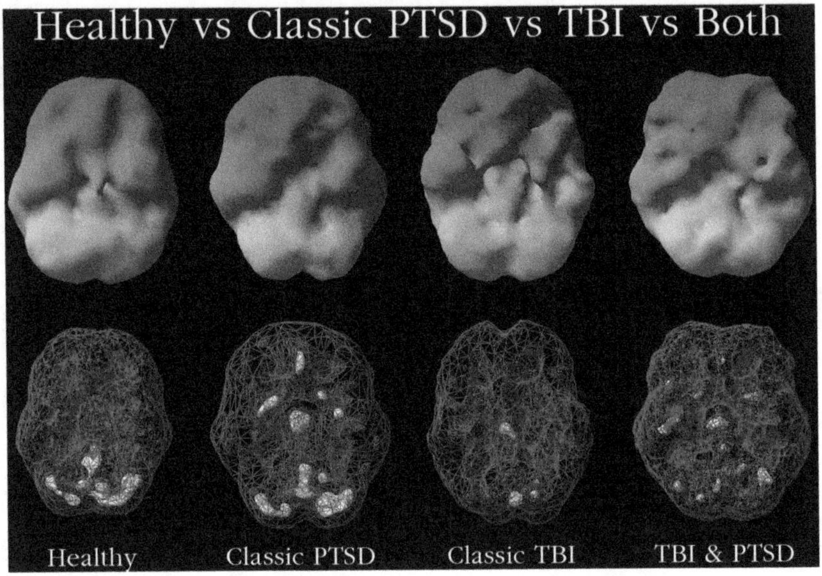


**Fig. 5.2** Brain SPECT Images of Healthy, PTSD, TBI and PTSD Co-morbid with TBI Perfusion Patterns

shows what a brain that has experienced PTSD looks like, compared with a 'healthy' brain, one that is not in a trauma response.

In the healthy brain, the two red areas show the stress hormone cortisol that's sitting at the base of the brain, where we would expect to see it. Cortisol is a hormone that is responsible for regulating processes that occur throughout the body, including how you metabolise your food, and immune responses. It also helps with motivation and activation and helps your body respond to stress[2] (Evans & Coccoma, 2014). The healthy brain is receiving a vast amount of information coming in from the brainstem, where there's a lot of activity going on. In contrast, in the brain experiencing PTSD, you can see that cortisol (in red), is dispersed throughout the whole of the brain.

[2] For a straightforward explanation of cortisol see https://www.webmd.com/a-to-z-guides/what-is-cortisol

It doesn't matter *where* information comes from, the whole system is ready to react. This is a brain that's on high alert, hypervigilant, looking for threat everywhere, ready to be retraumatised or retriggered. As it's always hyper-aroused, it goes easily into a fight or flight panic reaction. You have probably seen movies where the war veteran leaps for cover if a car backfires outside. That veteran's brain is still responding to the encoded threat stimulus of the bombs they experienced in the war. Brains experiencing PTSD have been pushed into a place where they're stuck in that high activation and can't return to the homeostasis that we talked about in Chap. 4. This brain knows that the world is not a safe place. It's not easy to pull all that dispersed cortisol back to get that brain out of activation, into a resting state where it can start to repair itself. This is why grounding and centring is so helpful in burning through that flooding cortisol.

A study by Ganzel et al. (2008) scanned the brains of healthy adults who had been within a mile and a half (2.4 km) of the attacks on the World Trade Centre on September 11, 2001. The study compared the scan results with healthy adults who had not been exposed to the 9/11 attacks. The main findings were that people who were closer to the attacks demonstrated more evidence of structural change in their brains following psychological trauma than people who were further away (Ganzel et al., 2008, p. 792). The brain scan images showed how trauma reduces the brain's grey matter in healthy adults who have been exposed to a traumatic event, as well as demonstrating how cortisol spreads throughout the PTSD brain.

We could also see this 9/11 example as a form of vicarious trauma (see Chap. 8). Seeing events like this happening in real time on TV, hearing about it or seeing it later on the news, could put us at risk of experiencing some degree of vicarious trauma. It could also be experienced as a collective trauma for people in the country that was attacked, or as a type of environmental trauma, which we turn to later in this chapter.

## Complex Trauma

In our experience, almost all traumas are complex. They not only activate your body, they also influence your mind, your relationships and how you view the world. To be considered complex trauma, a number of diagnostic criteria need to be present. First, the person must feel that the traumatic situation is *inescapable*, for example, in cases of domestic violence or child sexual abuse. Second, the trauma happens again and again; it is *repetitive*. Third, complex trauma is interpersonal; it happens *between people*. When the violation or the traumatic event happens between people, it impacts across a lot of systems, not just your worldview, your knowledge system, your physical system, but also your cognitions, how you think about things. Finally, complex trauma builds over time; it's *cumulative* (Herman, 2015).

In Chap. 4 we talked about what happens when the nervous system is continually activated; it can no longer come back to a resting state, it's always in activation, always in hyper-arousal. In those cases, your body makes adjustments, the way your *genes* are read can change (see the next section on epigenetics), your *brain* makes adjustments because it needs more cortisol to deal with the stress, rather than dopamine, the happy hormone. Think of a child who's in an abusive family situation that they can't escape. They're being exposed to stressful interactions between them and the perpetrator continually. Over time the child's nervous system makes adjustments as a response to that environment, placing the child in a continual threat response. Behaviours may look like not being able to sit still, play, or engage.

If someone's suffering complex trauma, it doesn't mean that they can't be affected by a single incident trauma or other unrelated traumas, the traumas just build up, layer upon layer. The brain experiencing PTSD we saw in Fig. 5.2, where the cortisol was spread throughout it, was a picture of a brain dealing with complex trauma. Situations of ongoing sexual abuse are almost always diagnosed as complex trauma because the whole system changes as it adjusts to the inescapable, repetitive and cumulative nature of that form of interpersonal abuse.

## Intergenerational Trauma and Epigenetics

We've been looking at how complex trauma can be cumulative. We might be tempted to think of that as happening to one person or people in a family, in one or two generations. But what if it continues to affect many generations? We call this *intergenerational trauma*. That is, each generation passes on to the next generation something different, not necessarily the exact same adaptive response to a threat, but the ability to survive the threat in a different way. The person's nervous system has made changes in order to survive and passes those changes to the next generation so *they* can survive, giving them a fighting chance.

We used to talk about *trans*generational trauma when we thought that trauma could be passed from one generation to their children. It is now known that trauma can be passed *down through multiple* generations, manifesting biologically, socially, psychologically, emotionally or environmentally. Consider this when you read the story about 'Murdering Creek Road' in Chap. 6.

In Australia, the impacts of historical events such as massacres and child removals, continue to be passed down through the generations. Colonisation continues today with ongoing systemic injury. The continual changing response of successive generations can be seen as intergenerational *resilience*. The impacts of historical trauma can have the effect of continuing 'the pathologizing of indigenous families' (Maxwell, 2014, p. 413), reinforcing a deficit rather than a strengths-based view of First Nations Peoples.

As a result of colonisation in Australia, as well as other countries that have been colonised by the British, such as New Zealand, Canada and North America, systemic racism, structural racism and racial trauma continue to affect Indigenous Peoples every day. (We yarn in more detail about racial trauma at the next billabong). Because of these systemic and structural realities, Indigenous Peoples continually experience a threat response. Not only do their bodies make adjustments, but the way their *genes* are read is adjusted.

The science of *epigenetics* explains the degree to which your genes are turned on or turned off in order to accommodate the environmental circumstances you live in. Before the growing interest in epigenetics, we used to believe that these changes were permanent. But we now know that's not true. According to current research, we understand that we *can* reverse those changes (Evans & Coccoma, 2014; Van der Kolk, 2014). We *can* repair the effects of ongoing and systemic racism resulting from colonisation.

In our training sessions, people often ask, "but how does trauma pass down through generations?" Since the earliest days of colonisation, Aboriginal and Torres Strait Islander Peoples who've become known as the 'Stolen Generations' in Australia (Wilson, 1997) have experienced being forcibly removed from their families. Many of those people who grew up in boarding schools, missions and children's homes were raised without the care of a loving parent, caregiver or community. For some of those people who never had the gift of loving families and parenting, they didn't have that to give to their children. An Elder who is a Stolen Generations survivor said to us, "don't use that word 'love', I don't know what that word means".

Epigenetics reveals another less obvious, but no less potent, form of intergenerational trauma. Our genes are not changed, but the way they are switched on or switched off, the way they are read, is what is changed by trauma (Carey, 2011). Therefore, this alteration is not genetic, but epigenetic. As Indigenous Peoples, our genes have made changes to help us survive the trauma of ongoing colonisation. From conception Indigenous children are being prepared for the ongoing reality they are about to be born into. As Aboriginal and Australian South Sea Island doctor, Mark Wenitong, said to us: "our babies come into this world born ready for the fight".

Some of the earliest work to come out of epigenetic studies has been about Holocaust survivors, which estimate that it could take about seven generations before the trauma of the Holocaust leaves the genetic systems of the families of survivors, as long as the threat has been removed (Danieli, 1985).

Don't be tempted to think of epigenetics and the changes to gene expression as a reason to pathologise; the body as a living system is making adjustments and adapting all the time. Like any coping behaviour, like any activation to minimise harm, you have to take account of the context in which it happens. The will to survive drives the coping behaviour. If the behaviour gives a positive outcome and we survive and thrive, our brains record the strategy and we use it again. This is resilience.

***Nicole***: *When I think about how we adjust to cope with the environment that we're born into, I remember looking at news reports in war zones, with bombs going off everywhere, and there are little children calmly sitting in the middle of it all. So maybe when they were developing in utero, they've learnt not to respond to big loud noises, which are part of their everyday environment.*

***Kelleigh***: *I think that's a really nice way to understand how it is for children who are sitting in the middle of war zones. They might be playing or talking to each other and you see people in uniform running around with protective headphones on, while these little bodies have just made adjustments. This environment has not been calm for a while. They've learnt and* *adjusted to tune out those noises. Changes in gene expression don't necessarily happen as a result of a single incident trauma, where one event doesn't always change you forever. It is an environmental change, an environmental need that causes your body to make an adaptation to stay alive.*

**Activity 5.4 The Healing Foundation Animation**

Take some time now to watch this beautiful animation[3] about healing from intergenerational trauma made by The Healing Foundation in Australia:

As you watch, reflect on these two questions:

What are two things that kept Aboriginal and Torres Strait Islander Peoples healthy before colonisation?

What do you think was the most damaging thing that came with the arrival of the tall ships? At the time of publication, this video had been suspended out of respect for Uncle Jack Charles, who had passed away recently, and his family. Uncle Jack Charles was a proud Boon Wurrung, Dja Dja Wurrung, Woiwurrung and Yorta Yorta man, a well-respected actor and activist, as well as a Stolen Generations survivor.

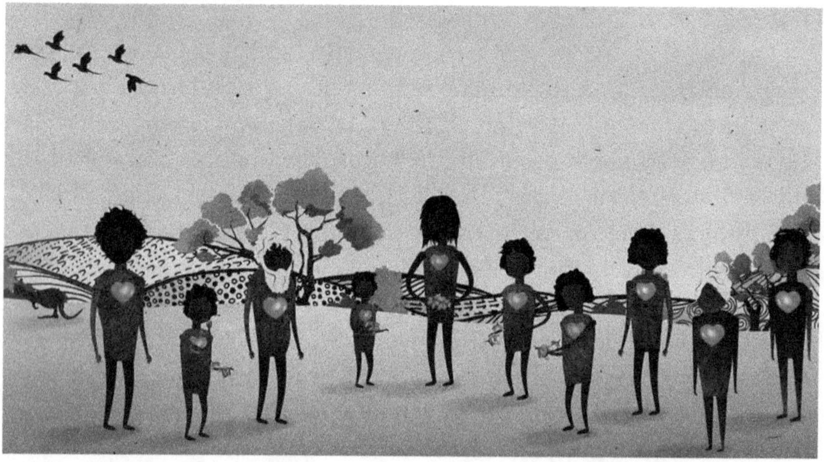

**Fig. 5.3** The Healing Foundation Intergenerational Trauma Animation

[3] https://www.youtube.com/watch?v=vlqx8EYvRbQ&feature=youtu.be&ab_channel=TheHealingFoundation

## Institutional Trauma

Institutional trauma is the trauma that arises from, as the name suggests, being forcibly separated from community and family and placed into institutions like children's' homes, residential schools and missions run by churches, and the mistreatment and abuse suffered by so many Indigenous people in these places. Understanding the legacy of this type of trauma is not only important for us here in Australia, but also for many First Nations Peoples around the world who experienced similar removals of thousands of children from their families and communities.

While there are similarities with intergenerational trauma, there are features of institutional trauma that are quite distinctive and, in some ways, considerably more damaging. These have been well documented in the reports of the *National Inquiry into the Separation of Aboriginal and Torres Strait Islander Children from Their Families* (Wilson, 1997); the *Royal Commission into Institutional Responses to Child Sexual Abuse* (McClellan, et al., 2017) and the Canadian *Royal Commission into Aboriginal Peoples* (Dussault et al., 1996).

One of the most damaging legacies of institutional trauma is 'institutional betrayal' (Smith & Freyd, 2013). Abuse was rife in the kinds of institutions Indigenous children were forced into. Many of the perpetrators of this abuse, the 'bad apples', the offenders, were just moved along, never punished for their crimes. The umbrella of the institution itself keeps the perpetrators nameless and 'punishless', keeping them above the law, beyond reproach. Many victims have never had their experiences recognised or validated. It's like an institutional silencing or denial that anything was ever wrong, that any crimes were committed. The leaders and managers of these institutions often covered things up, moved the perpetrators around, seemingly oblivious to, or not caring about, the traumatising effects of their actions on the individual children in their care. The responsibility lies with the system, which responds by either removing or adjusting or 'managing' the problem. It's very different when you can engage with someone face to face and hold them responsible for their actions.

When Institutional betrayal also includes unwanted sexual experiences, people often have more dissociative symptoms (Smith & Freyd, 2014). A likely explanation is that in situations like kids in children's homes, or adults in mental health institutions, where people can't escape, have no power, and don't have a voice, the only way they can remove themselves from that pain and the trauma that's being acted out on them, is to take their consciousness away and disconnect. That's the last choice available to their brains.

Remember we're not talking about children being removed because they were neglected and taken to an environment where they were given great food and looked after and cared for and loved. But that is still a prevalent belief we hear time and again in non-Indigenous Australia. You'll still hear people say when they hear of Aboriginal and Torres Strait Islander children being taken to children's homes or residential schools, "but they were much better off being there than where they came from".

Another misconception that reflects the lack of understanding of institutional trauma is people often believe that when you take the child or the adult out of the institution that they'll just 'get over it'. They don't realise that all that systemic abuse still needs to be healed. Removing the threat only minimises *future* abuse.

## Institutional Trauma at the Kinchela Boys Home

This is a picture of some of the Elders who are survivors of the Kinchela Boys Home (KBH) (Fig. 5.4), a home set up in 1924 and not closed until 1970. It was built on the stolen land of the *Dunghutti* people near Kempsey, New South Wales. Hundreds of young Aboriginal boys, some as young as 6 weeks old, were sent there over those many years, after being forcibly removed from their families. These are men who are part of an organisation called the Kinchela Boys Aboriginal Corporation (KBHAC), who want their stories to be told. Our organisation, *The Seedling Group*, has done a lot of careful work and knowledge sharing with the men of the KBHAC.

'The Kinchela Boys', as they call themselves, were told that their parents didn't love them, or that their parents had died; they had all of their clothes

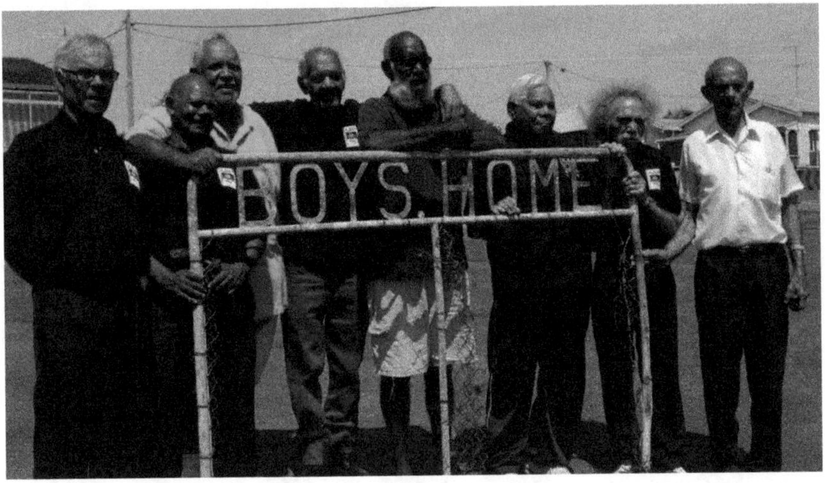


**Fig. 5.4** Kinchela Boys Home survivors. With permission from KBHAC

removed and burned, and all of their papers burned. They were not called by their names, but were referred to only by a number. So even today, when we meet with them, they'll say, "Number 28? Yeah, he was there that day." Every part of their identity, including their culture, was taken away from them. The institution was known for its sexual abuse, and children were chained to a tree out in the dark as punishment. That tree, to this day, still has a couple of the links of that chain within its trunk; the tree is gradually growing over that chain. We are *not* talking here about kids who were removed and put into a 'better place'. We are talking about systematic, horrifying institutional abuse and its resulting trauma.

Those traumas are ongoing. Now these men have been doing amazing work, building a resource that is *interrupting* that intergenerational and institutional trauma. When the men learned about trauma and its effects, it was a complete game changer for them, giving them back so much power. This is why we feel it's important this information gets out to people who have had trauma in their lives, whether they're Indigenous or non-Indigenous.[4]

[4] See more about what the men of the KBHAC are doing on their website https://kinchelaboyshome.org.au/

## Collective Trauma

In Australia, colonisation has brought widespread and ongoing collective trauma for Aboriginal and Torres Strait Islander Peoples. Fundamentally flawed historical and current government policies continue to impact on multiple peoples across multiple generations. Huge numbers of Aboriginal people were removed from their communities, taken from their Nations, out of their language groups where they had their own lore, their own marriage rules, their own songlines, trading routes, rituals and ceremonies. People from different Nations were forced to live together in government and church-controlled places like reserves or missions. They were expected to live as one homogenous race. Removal often meant the loss of cultural practices, reciprocal relationships, kinship lines and connections. Connections acknowledge relationships to each other, the spirit of rivers, mountains, and all entities of Country, totems, neighbouring Nations and trading lines across time. These are what make you part of a community, make you a family, help you function and give you identity and purpose. Expecting community or those relationships to recover by themselves, is unrealistic.

The term 'collective trauma' was first used in the literature by psychiatrist Kai Erikson (1976) to describe a man-made flooding disaster on the small mining communities of Buffalo Creek in the United States, in which 125 people died (Krieg, 2009, p. S29). Erikson recognised how important it is to:

> distinguish between collective and individual experiences of trauma in order to underscore the difficulty for people to recover from the effects of individual trauma when the community on which they have depended has become fragmented and disconnected (Krieg, 2009, p. S29).

What he saw was a community that had been completely wiped out. And when the people from the community started coming back, what was apparent was that the relationships that had always been in that community had broken down. All those simple things that make us a community, all those relationships, and all the knowing that we have between ourselves, were missing. The Holocaust is another example of collective trauma, where families had to out other families for being Jewish (Danieli, 1985). Families turned on other families in their community. These were people who had been living in harmony, people who had been in communities and villages caring for each other before the Holocaust changed everything. Much of that connection broke down.

This extraordinary yet haunting map (Fig. 5.5) shows the different communities from which each of the Kinchela boys was removed between 1924 and 1969. Take a moment now to reflect on the impact that the removal of their children had on all of those communities. Some Aboriginal communities had *all* of the children removed within a few years. We've heard Stolen Generations people saying, "we feel so much for our parents because suddenly there were no children; there was no one to hand the stories down to; there was no one to hand our traditions down to; they were all just gone." For an oral storytelling culture, this was the fracturing of identity of our cultural connections on an unimaginable scale.

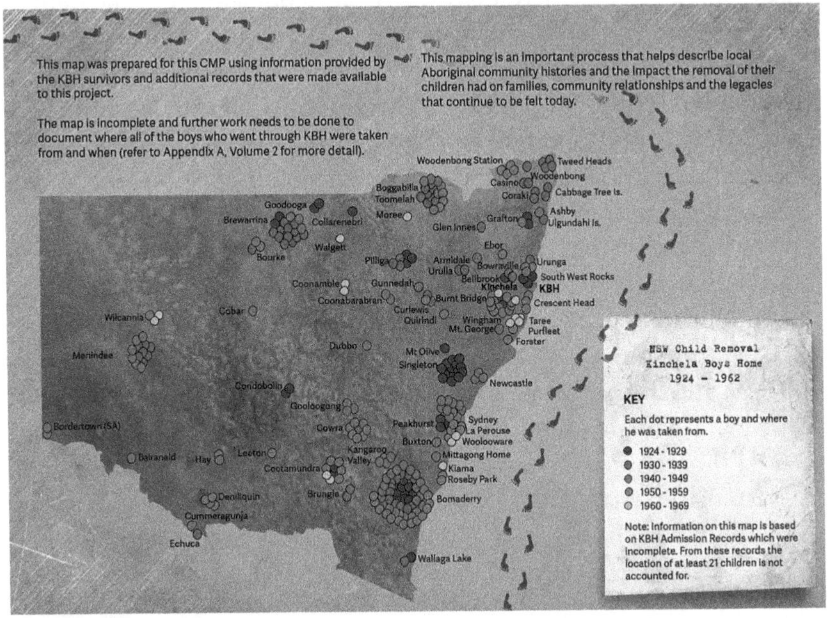


**Fig. 5.5** Map of Kinchela Boys Home removals. Source: Kinchela Boys' Home Aboriginal Corporation (2017, p. 5), with permission

Think of someone coming and taking your child away, for no other reason than the colour of their skin, and them believing that you're just going to get over it; that it's not going to affect you; that it's not going to affect your family, your children. It has, in fact, had a *catastrophic* impact. While First Nations families did everything they could to fight for their children, they had no legal avenues to battle the injustice of the policies at that time. It affected people, not just in behaviours, not just in cognitions and beliefs, it affected them on a deep, cellular level. So many of our people, mothers and fathers, just died of broken hearts. We pay our respects to those who lost their lives and families in the fight to reclaim their children.

## Historical Trauma

Australia is made up of different peoples with different history stories. For us, the many Nations of Indigenous Australia, our history stories began long before the arrival of the British to our shores. In the fullness of time, colonised Australia is but a blip on our history timeline.

Archaeologists have found the places where our families gathered and lived in 60,000 BC. We have long history stories on this continent. See The Healing Foundation timeline[5] to see major events of this story. What is your history story and when does it intersect ours?

From the arrival of the British to this continent in 1788 up until the 1950s, the population of First Nations Peoples declined from an estimated 750,000 to 70,000 (Pocock, 2008). This decline can be attributed to a combination of early colonial warfare, government-sanctioned massacres, introduced diseases, famine, and genocidal policies (Reynolds, 2001). A full list of the massacre sites in Australia can be found on the Australian Museum website.[6] Historical trauma in Australia was formalised through making laws that allowed the removal and destruction of Australia's First Nations Peoples, intending them to be 'bred out' (McGregor, 2002), all as part of the colonial governing system.

---

[5] https://healingfoundation.org.au/timeline-trauma-healing-australia/

[6] australian.museum

Knowing your culture is a protective factor, no matter where you come from in the world. Other protective factors of cultural identity include language, laws, ways of being, cultural rituals and ceremonies, religion, presence on land, or knowing where and to whom you belong. We know that people who have been separated from their land, such as refugees and people seeking asylum, people who have been a long time without having a country, fare worse than those who still have a country they can connect to and which gives them identity (Akinyemi et al., 2012).

In Australia, protective factors were destroyed when children were stolen, and any trace of their culture removed, when people were forcibly moved off their traditional lands, and discriminating Government policies were enacted with purposeful and destructive intent. This deep hurt lives in our communities today and is reinforced by practices that dismiss our histories. This is historical trauma.

An easy way to understand this is the different ways that Invasion Day is celebrated in Australia. In the mainstream history story, Invasion Day is labelled Australia Day.

Nicole: *When I teach undergraduate students about Invasion Day, it is the foreign students who are horrified when they learn what they are celebrating when they join into Australia Day celebrations. Many young Australian students are also confused when they reflect upon the conflicting messages about why Australia Day is celebrated. It has been one of those holidays that people celebrate without questioning too much.*

While Australia day continues to celebrate milestones in the colonisation of us, it continues to deepen our historical trauma wounds which show up in our communities today as over representation in the justice system, alarming suicide rates and persistent health disparities. For us, it is more important to use the day to fight for the recognition of our true history story and those who came before us who fought to make that story known. This truth telling, and moving this truth telling into the collective consciousness of Australia, is a fundamental step towards our healing from historical trauma.

Now that we have yarned about historical trauma, lets contemplate how that would impact our day to day culturally safe trauma-informed practice. When you ask someone 'who's your mob?' what are you really asking that person? How will their answer change, if anything, the way you interact and have a working relationship with them?

When thinking back to the principles of trauma-informed practice; *safety, trustworthiness, choice, collaboration, empowerment, and culture,* think about how the historical trauma story of a person or community would influence the way you work. Is there more you need to know, who could you collaborate with to make sure you are as informed as you can be? What does safety look like for that community or that family when you understand the historical trauma story?

Nicole: *For example, if I am working in a community that was colonised by missionaries, I am conscious about asking where the appropriate place to meet might be. A church hall might be a triggering place for some families. The historical trauma of every community is different and affects how I will work there, and it is my responsibility to learn the story of that community so that I can work there with safety.*

The next section gives more detail about what has been written about historical trauma in different countries, to give you more perspective on the global nature of this pervasive and challenging type of trauma. If historical trauma seems to have overlapping concepts with intergenerational trauma and other traumas, you are not mistaken. The next section gives you more detailed analysis of the subtle differences that researchers have given to the different types of trauma.

Want to know more about historical trauma?

**Introduction**

When we talk about historical trauma, we all know that bad stuff that happened in the past still affects our mob today. We don't really need reminding that colonisation is at the root of so many of the issues we continue to face on a daily basis. It started with Captain Cook claiming Aboriginal land for the British Crown in 1770, declaring it *terra nullius* (literally, 'empty land') and it hasn't stopped.

When we delve a bit deeper into research done in this field, mainly by psychiatrists, psychologists, health researchers, legal practitioners and historians, it becomes apparent that not only have Indigenous peoples across the world had similar experiences, but a range of definitions and terms are used to describe the impact of historical trauma on other oppressed groups as well.

(*continued*)

**(continued)**

The term 'historical trauma' was first used in relation to ongoing trauma experienced by survivors and descendants of the Jewish Holocaust in Nazi Germany in the second World War (Danieli, 1985). The term has since been used to describe suffering of a range of different ethnic groups around the globe, for example, descendants of the legacy of African slavery in America, descendants of the Japanese American internment camps during World War II, descendants of the Khmer Rouge violence in Cambodia in the 1970s and descendants of Maya refugees from the 1980s Guatemalan genocide (Hatala et al., 2015).

A number of researchers point out the differences between the Holocaust and Indigenous historical trauma. For example, North American scholars argue that while there are some similarities, a significant difference between the Jewish experiences of the 1930s and 1940s and those of Native Americans is the sense that the initial trauma was not confined to a single catastrophic period: over a period of 400 years, Native Americans "experienced one of the most systematic and successful programs of ethnic cleansing the world has seen" (Whitbeck et al., 2004, p. 121).

Our focus here is how the concept of historical trauma, and other similar terms, have been applied to Aboriginal peoples subjected to colonisation in Canada, Australia, New Zealand and the United States, sometimes referred to as the CANZUS nations (Paradies, 2016, p. 85). Australian health researcher Karen Menzies recently published a literature review that explores the history of the concept and its relevance for Australian Aboriginal experience (Menzies, 2019). You might find it a good place to start to get the lay of the land for this topic.

**Definitions of historical trauma**

The term was first applied to Aboriginal peoples in North America in the 1990s by Lakota woman Maria Yellow Horse Brave Heart (1998) and Duran & Duran (1995). Brave Heart defines historical trauma as the "cumulative emotional and psychological wounding, over the lifespan and across generations, emanating from massive group trauma experiences" (as cited in Hatala et al., 2015, p. 1913).

Bringing the different interpretations and definitions together, the main elements that distinguish historical trauma include: an *initial trauma* or 'wounding' *perpetrated by outsiders with purposeful and often destructive intent,* which is *shared by a group* of people, spanning *multiple generations,* generating high levels of *distress and mourning in present day communities, reinforced through ongoing racism and discrimination* (Evans-Campbell, 2008; Mohatt et al., 2014; Gone, 2013).

(*continued*)

**(continued)**

Indigenous psychiatrist Professor Helen Milroy offers this description of the multi-layered effects of historical/intergenerational trauma on Aboriginal and Torres Strait Islander peoples, which occur:

> via a variety of mechanisms including the impact of attachment relationships with care givers; the impact on parenting and family functioning; the association with parental physical and mental illness; disconnection and alienation from the extended family, culture and society. These effects are exacerbated by exposure to continuing high levels of stress and trauma including multiple bereavements and other losses, the process of vicarious traumatisation where children witness the on-going effects of the original trauma which a parent or care giver has experienced. Even where children are protected from the traumatic stories of their ancestors, the effects of past traumas still impact on children in the form of ill health, family dysfunction, community violence, psychological morbidity and early mortality (as cited in Menzies, 2019, p. 1527).

**Similar terms, different definitions**

When you start reading in this area, you'll find that scholars and researchers use the term 'historical trauma' interchangeably with other terms, such as 'soul wound', collective unresolved grief, collective trauma, intergenerational trauma, transgenerational trauma, intergenerational posttraumatic stress, multigenerational trauma (Reid & Varona, 2014, p. 518). Others use terms such as 'cultural trauma' (Halloran, 2004) and 'frozen trauma' (Davoine & Gaudilliere, 2004).

Some argue that historical trauma is distinct from intergenerational trauma in that "intergenerational trauma refers to the specific experience of trauma across familial generations, but does not necessarily imply a shared group trauma. Similarly, a collective trauma may not have the generational or historical aspect, though over time may develop into historical trauma" (Mohatt et al., 2014).

Australian psychologist Michael Halloran uses the term 'cultural trauma' to describe the:

> interruption of cultural knowledge and practices in order to undermine the worth of a people... which [in Australia] included land dispossession by force, theft of women, slavery and war, introduced diseases,

(*continued*)

**(continued)**

and the missionary zeal for Aboriginal people to embrace Western religion and reject their own spiritual beliefs such as the dreaming. Moreover, settlement brought with it the assertion of British sovereignty and law, which effectively displaced indigenous customary law (Halloran, 2004, p. 5).

Davoine and Gaudilliere (2004) use the term 'frozen trauma' to explain how past trauma can remain present and describe "the impact of cultural genocide, geographic displacement or forced removal as a 'dehistoricization of experience'" (as cited in Menzies, 2019, p. 1526).

**Individual/biological vs collective focus: differences with PTSD**

Many people writing about historical trauma are keen to make the distinction between the collective experience of historical trauma and the more individual one of post traumatic stress disorder (PTSD). Joseph Gone, a Native American professor of psychology and member of the *Aaniiih-Gros Ventre* tribal nation, sees historical trauma as "a counterbalance to the increasing prevalence of biological explanations for mental health problems" as it "accentuates and implicates the processes of colonization rather than faulty genes or broken brains". He argues that by taking a relational rather than an individual perspective, historical trauma "links community members together in shared struggles to overcome bitter circumstance or frightful ordeal in the wake of colonisation", believing that traditional Indigenous approaches have the potential to mitigate the cumulative, intergenerational impacts of historical trauma (Gone, 2013, p. 688).

Australian mental health worker Anthea Krieg, who has lived in and worked with remote and urban Aboriginal communities for more than 25 years, argues that "the inappropriateness of a PTSD diagnosis for collective experience is becoming increasingly apparent." She says that while Aboriginal people identify with the concept of historical trauma as it acknowledges and provides a context for ongoing injustice, "it risks being misappropriated into the psychiatric realm of PTSD" (Krieg, 2009, p. S30).

**The flipside: 'historical privilege'**

We conclude with an interesting 'flip' from Aotearoa New Zealand (Borell et al., 2018). These authors argue that a similar logic that applies to historical *trauma* experienced by Indigenous people and their descendants should be applied to the other side of the coin, the historical *privilege* that accrues to 'settlers' and their descendants. They come up with the following

*(continued)*

**(continued)**

'working definition' of historical privilege to test this construction: "The complex and collective structural advantages experienced over time and across generations by a group of people who share an identity, affiliation, or circumstance" (p. 26).

The authors frame the context in this way (the parallels with the Australian context are pretty clear!):

> The Pākehā [white] settlers who acquired the land and material resources taken from Māori have reaped individual, collective and intergenerational rewards from that procurement. The accumulated effects over generations have dramatically improved the economic, social and political wellbeing of current descendants, both materially and structurally. Pākehā worldviews and the institutionalisation of Pākehā cultural norms in our national, governmental and civic institutions have served to reaffirm and entrench models of mental and social wellbeing (Borell et al., 2018, p. 26).

They go on to demonstrate how the key elements of historical trauma can be 'flipped' to apply to historical privilege. Here is a summary based on a table the authors provide. You can read the paper for the specific details and see how they align (or not) with the Australian context and experience:

**Key elements of historical trauma and historical privilege**

| Key elements | Historical trauma | Historical privilege |
|---|---|---|
| Acts of trauma | Acts of trauma experienced through colonisation | Acts of historic windfall and dramatic increases in wealth, power and social status |
| Ongoing renewal of historical acts | Recurring experiences of racism discrimination | Naturalisation of group superiority through structural, institutional & cultural favouritism |
| Experienced by a group/collective | Affected groups may share a particular identity, affiliation or circumstance | Individual and familial wealth acquisition supported by government action |
| Experienced by multiple generations | Trauma affecting multiple generations of descendants who may not have witnessed the original act(s) themselves | Historic boons in wealth, power and social status are passed to and added on by subsequent generations of settlers |
| Remembrance/forgetting | Remembrance and commemoration are inherent with an underlying importance on healing, resilience and recompense | Collective forgetting is more common. Remembrance is carefully constructed (e.g. ANZAC commemorations) |

Source: Borell et al. (2018, p. 31)

The paper concludes: "If we are serious about addressing the ill effects of colonisation on one population, equitable acknowledgement of the privileging effects consequential to another must also be part of the conversation" (p. 31).

**Activity 5.5 Reflective Questions on Historical Trauma**

- How useful is the concept of historical trauma to your everyday life and work?
- How much do you know about the early experiences of your ancestors, whether you are Indigenous or non-Indigenous?
- What terms and definitions make most sense to you?
- How applicable do you think the concept of 'historical privilege' is to the Australian context?
- How would you go about having a conversation with others about the concepts of historical trauma and historical privilege?

## Environmental Trauma

We end this chapter where we started. The first trauma for Aboriginal and Torres Strait Islander Peoples was environmental trauma when lands were taken by the British under the pretext of *terra nullius* (empty land). This next section goes into more detail about how environmental trauma has impacted on First Nations Peoples across the world, from the taking of land in early colonial times to environmental injustices with land being degraded, mined and poisoned, through to the current ever-present trauma and vulnerability to climate change.

### Want to Know More About Environmental Trauma?

Loss of connection to traditional lands and country has been described by some authors as 'place-based environmental historical trauma' (Beltrán, Schultz, Fernandez, & Evans-Campbell, 2018), demonstrating the strong links between historical acts of colonisation and current day environmental trauma. Place-based environmental historical trauma also links loss of country to loss of collective spiritual health and identity (p. 104).

While you won't find much reference to the term 'environmental trauma' in the literature, '*environmental justice*' is a term that often relates to injustices towards First Nations Peoples in relation to degradation and poisoning of land through contamination (Green, 2017; Hanlon, 2008; Kenney, 2012; Newell, 2005; Shriver & Webb, 2009; Wiebe, 2016) and activities such as mining taking priority over Indigenous rights to land

and livelihood (Brugge & Goble, 2002; Gundjehmi Aboriginal Corporation, n.d.; Marsh & Green, 2020; Necefer et al., 2015).

While not discussed in terms of trauma, these examples leave no doubt that the experiences of First Nations Peoples in fighting for land justice could be described as environmental trauma. In Australia, the impact of mining in particular has taken a huge toll. The world knows about the travesty of the destruction in May 2020 of sites sacred to the Puutu Kunti Kurrama and Pinikura Peoples at Juukan Gorge in Western Australia by mining company Rio Tinto (Wensing, 2020). However, little is known about the unrelenting pressure on Traditional Owners when they 'negotiated' with uranium mining companies in the Northern Territory in the 1970s. Hear the voice of one Traditional Owner in this extract from a letter written in 1977:

> Everyone is pushing us. Pushing, pushing, pushing. Now they want us to sign but they don't know what it means for us. This is our life… I'll ask you one question. How much is your life worth? How much do I have to pay you so I can take your life away? People will say that we are just trying to make trouble now and stop everything, but we don't want trouble. We just want you to understand what we are giving up … our life. …
>
> We don't know what is wrong with you. We are always straight with you. but now we must do something ourselves. We have seen what happened to others when mining came too quickly. They've lost. They're getting skinny. They don't believe in that mining any more. We don't want that to happen to us and so we have asked for our stories to be written (Gundjehmi Aboriginal Corporation, n.d., p. 37).

In the United States and Canada, First Nations Peoples have been fighting similar injustices since colonisation (Vickery & Hunter, 2016). A long and interesting paper by Brett Clark (2002) analyses and describes some of the ongoing campaigns of the Indigenous Environmental Movement in the US, in particular those of the Chippewa (against mining companies), the Mohawk (against pollution of land and water from industrialisation), and the Western Shoshone (against uranium mining). He concludes with quoting Shoshone poet Silko, who wrote in 1996:

> This is no new war. This war has a five-hundred-year history. This is the same war of resistance that the indigenous people of the Americas have never ceased to fight ... We are all part of the old stories. Whether we know the stories or not, the stories know about us (as cited in Clark, 2002, p. 430).

As a result of these hundreds of years of colonisation, land degradation, mining and pollution, the world now faces the reality of the impacts of a rapidly changing climate. And it is us, the world's First Nations Peoples, who are feeling these impacts on the frontline. It is the Inuit peoples, whose traditional livelihoods are directly threatened by the loss of sea ice (Cunsolo Willox & Ellis, 2018; Durkalec et al., 2015); it is the Saami peoples, the Indigenous people who live in the northern parts of Norway, Sweden, Finland, and Russia (Jaakkola et al., 2018); it is the peoples of the Canadian arctic where thinning sea ice prevents them from engaging with glaciers as spiritual entities (Allison, 2015); it is the many peoples of the Pacific Islands, like the people from Tuvalu, a coral atoll nation, who are under extreme psychological stress as sea levels rise around them (Gibson et al., 2020); and it is the peoples of the Torres Strait, who live only two metres above sea level and who have been advocating in vain at the highest levels for recognition of the vulnerability of their peoples, and all Indigenous peoples, to the impacts of climate change (Hunter, 2009).

In 2008, Aboriginal and Torres Strait Islander delegates on climate change addressed the United Nations Permanent Forum on Indigenous Issues in New York:

> Madam Chair, climate change raises distinct challenges for Indigenous peoples, our cultures and our lands and resources. It poses a threat to the health, cultures and livelihoods of Indigenous peoples. This occurs in coastal and flood prone areas, salt inundation of freshwater supplies, changes to mangroves and fire regimes, coastal erosion and rising sea levels as well as for those Indigenous communities affected by long term drought and desertification, among other impacts (Hunter, 2009, p. 445).

In their recommendations, the delegation emphasised the need for full participation of Indigenous Peoples and respect for Indigenous cultural knowledge and law in designing mitigation measures to ensure that:

> such measures do not contribute to the further dispossession of Indigenous people from our land and resources, or impact adversely on the cultural traditions, languages, traditional knowledge and traditional food sources of Indigenous communities (Hunter, 2009, p. 446).

Years later, the words of those delegates have still gone unheeded. In some islands in the Torres Strait, rising sea levels have exposed the bones of their ancestors.

There are plenty of studies and research done into the impact of climate change on Indigenous mental health, which you may be interested to investigate (Berry et al., 2008; Berry et al., 2018; Boyd & Parr, 2020; Cunsolo Willox & Ellis, 2018; Ford, 2012; Gibson et al., 2020; Johnson et al., 2021; McNamara & Westoby, 2011; Middleton et al., 2020; Pearce et al., 2015; Petheram et al., 2015; Petheram et al., 2010; Rigby et al., 2011; Williams, 2012).

To finish up this section, we leave you with some Aboriginal and Torres Strait Islander voices, reflecting on the impacts of climate change on their social and emotional wellbeing. We start with reflections from three Aunties from Erub Island in the Torres Strait, who spoke to researchers Karen McNamara & Ross Westoby (2011, p. 235):

> We live on the island surrounded by sea, and I took my artwork from here and the land… The tide is getting higher now. We used to have the shells. There's not much now. We used to go out and collect octopus but it's really hard now to find octopus and for the shell as well, like clam shell or spider shell; it's really hard.
>
> We used to read the landscape. But now it changes, you have to guess now. … Like before, you can know what's gonna happen. So hard now, guessing all the time … I think it start changing in the 1980s, the changes start… Am sad at home, think about the good old days, we always talk about the good old days. Now everything is changing, even the trees, you can see changes in them, even the fruits, like before, we haven't had mango season.
>
> When I was young we used to go further out on the beach, the beach was right out… But now, it change a lot and the water comes right in, right up to the back door, I mean, my laundry and the back step in the house… We used to walk all the way out to where the rocks are. Yeah, we can't do that anymore… If it's going to still come in, up to the house and that, where would I go? I would have to leave all of my life at the house but I don't want to.

Petheram et al. (2010) ran workshops and in-depth interviews in two coastal *Yolngu* Aboriginal communities, Yirrkala and Wallaby Beach, in East Arnhem Land (Northern Territory). The researchers went there to ask people about what they thought about climate change, what they had been noticing and what they thought should be done to adapt to the changes. Many, especially younger men, emphasised the extreme differences between *Yolngu* and '*Balanda*' (non-Indigenous) worldviews:

> We see the land through painting, stories, songs, totem lines. Balanda don't understand how Yolngu connect and relate to the land … They see totally opposite. They see career, money and future… They are wiping out our identity and our minds (p. 683).

When talking about the power of the Rio Tinto bauxite mine they have had to live with since the 1970s:

> … they are digging up the backbone of the Yolngu … the mine is like a big mob of sharks coming in when the tide is out … It's like you can't get out of the water, it's stopping you (p. 685).

When talking about what changes the men were seeing:

> In some areas turtles no longer come to nest—they are confused with the erosion and changes … [the seasonal calendar] is all mixed up … the wet season is late this year…we are hot and we are waiting …why is it so hot now?' [Kangaroos, emus, certain snakes] are harder to find …we have to go further for hunting [Green plum tree flowers normally indicate that] sting rays are fat and ready to eat … right now they are flowering and the rays are not ready… Since we were children we have seen big changes. In the time the changes have already happened and they are here—we are trying to deal with it and trying to be strong (p. 686).

Women were more likely to mention 'intuitive' changes:

> We can sense something…there is also this strange roaring in the water – I've never heard that. I don't know what it is …Spirits are visiting people in dreams more often' (p. 686).

## Concluding Comments

Understanding the different types of trauma helps us appreciate the many layers of trauma that people can be carrying. With this understanding, it is possible to trace the origins of social and health disparities affecting priority populations. It also provides an insight into social bias and stereotyping that manifest in expressions of covert and overt racism. The next billabong talks about how racial trauma is deeply embedded in our society, and the reality of this for Indigenous Peoples. Before we move to that next chapter, take a few moments to ground yourself, check out and reflect.

**Activity 5.6 Grounding Exercise**

A simple way to move your muscle groups is to shake your legs. Stand up and do this now. You can also ground yourself simply by humming, singing, or raising your voice to the ancestors, all of which are sensory motor exercises that massage your Vagus nerve. You many want to spend a minute reflecting on the First Nations Peoples whose land you are living on and benefiting from and thank them for their custodianship.

**Activity 5.7 Check out and Reflection**

Take a moment to check out. Do a scan of your body and sense how you're feeling and where you feel it after coming to the end of this very big chapter. Then write some answers to these reflective questions:

- What was the main thing you learned from this chapter that will stay with you?
- What information challenged you most?
- What do you think are the main differences between intergenerational, collective and historical trauma?
- What was something new you learned in the section on environmental trauma?
- How will you use the knowledge you've taken from this billabong?
- What difference could this knowledge make to your family and community life?

## References and Further Reading

Aboriginal and Torres Strait Islander Healing Foundation. (2019). *Timeline of Trauma and Healing in Australia*. Retrieved from https://healingfoundation.org.au/timeline-trauma-healing-australia/

Akinyemi, O. O., Owoaje, E. T., Ige, O. K., & Popoola, O. A. (2012). Comparative study of mental health and quality of life in long term refugees and host populations in Oru-Ijebu, Southwest Nigeria. *BMC Research Notes, 5*(1), 1–9.

Allen, R. E., & Oliver, J. M. (1982). The effects of child maltreatment on language development. *Child Abuse and Neglect, 6*, 299–305.

Allison, E. A. (2015). The spiritual significance of glaciers in an age of climate change. *Wiley Interdisciplinary Reviews: Climate Change, 6*(5), 493–508.

Amen, D. G., Raji, C. A., Willeumier, K., Taylor, D., Tarzwell, R., Newberg, A., & Henderson, T. A. (2015). Functional neuroimaging distinguishes posttraumatic stress disorder from traumatic brain injury in focused and large community datasets. *PLoS One, 10*(7). https://doi.org/10.1371/journal.pone.0129659

Atkinson, S., & Swain, S. (1999). A network of support: Mothering across the Koorie community in Victoria, Australia. *Women's History Review, 8*(2), 219–230.

Bartholomew, K., & Horowitz, L. M. (1991). Attachment styles among young adults: A test of a four-category model. *Journal of Personality and Social Psychology, 61*(2), 226–244. https://doi.org/10.1037/0022-3514.61.2.226

Beckett, C., Maughan, B., Rutter, M., Castle, J., Colvert, E., Groothues, C., Kreppner, J., Stevens, S., O'Connor, T. G., & Sonuga-Barke, E. J. S. (2006). Do the effects of early severe deprivation on cognition persist into early adolescence? Findings from the English and Romanian Adoptees study. *Child Development, 77*(3), 696–711. https://doi.org/10.1111/j.1467-8624.2006.00898.x

Beltrán, R., Schultz, K., Fernandez, A. R., & Evans-Campbell, T. (2018). From ambivalence to revitalization: Negotiating cardiovascular health behaviors related to environmental and historical trauma in a Northwest American Indian community. *American Indian and Alaska Native Mental Health Research, 25*(2), 103–128.

Berry, H. L., Kelly, B. J., Hanigan, I. C., Coates, J. H., McMichael, A. J., Welsh, J. A., & Kjellstrom, T. (2008). *Rural mental health impacts of climate change: Commissioned report for the Garnaut Climate Change Review*. Retrieved from Canberra

Berry, H. L., Waite, T. D., Dear, K. B. G., Capon, A. G., & Murray, V. (2018). The case for systems thinking about climate change and mental health. *Nature Climate Change, 8*(4), 282–290.

Bombay, A., Matheson, K., & Anisman, H. (2013). The intergenerational effects of Indian Residential Schools: Implications for the concept of historical trauma. *Transcultural Psychiatry, 51*(3), 320–338.

Borell, B., Moewaka Barnes, H., & McCreanor, T. (2018). Conceptualising historical privilege: The flip side of historical trauma, a brief examination. *AlterNative: An International Journal of Indigenous Peoples, 14*(1), 25–34.

Bowlby, J. (1988). *A secure base: Parent-child attachment and healthy human development.* Basic Books.

Boyd, C., & Parr, H. (2020). Climate change and rural mental health: A geographic perspective. *Rural and Remote Health, 20*(4), 6337. https://doi.org/10.22605/RRH6337

Brave Heart, M. Y. H. (1998). The return to the sacred path: Healing the historical trauma and historical unresolved grief response among the Lakota through a psychoeducational group intervention. *Smith College Studies in Social Work, 68*(3), 287–305.

Bretherton, I. (1992). The origins of attachment theory: John Bowlby and Mary Ainsworth. *Developmental Psychology, 28*(5), 759–775.

Brugge, D., & Goble, R. (2002). The history of uranium mining and the Navajo People. *American Journal of Public Health, 92*(9), 1410–1419. https://doi.org/10.2105/AJPH.92.9.1410

Buchheim, A., George, C., Gündel, H., & Viviani, R. (2017). Neuroscience of human attachment. *Frontiers in Human Neuroscience, 11*, 1–136. https://doi.org/10.3389/fnhum.2017.00136

Carey, N. (2011). *The epigenetics revolution.* Icon Books.

Carriere, J., & Richardson, C. (2009). From longing to belonging: Attachment theory, connectedness, and Indigenous children in Canada. In S. Mckay, D. Fuchs, & I. Brown (Eds.), *Passion for action in child and family services: Voices from the Prairies* (pp. 49–67). Canadian Plains Research Centre.

Choate, P. W., Kohler, T., Cloete, F., CrazyBull, B., Lindstrom, D., & Tatoulis, P. (2019). Rethinking Racine v Woods from a decolonizing perspective: Challenging the applicability of attachment theory to Indigenous families involved with child protection. *Canadian Journal of Law and Society / Revue Canadienne Droit et Société, 34*(1), 55–78.

Clark, B. (2002). The Indigenous environmental movement in the United States: Transcending borders in struggles against mining, manufacturing, and

the capitalist state. *Organization & Environment, 15*(4), 410–442. https://doi.org/10.1177/1086026602238170
Cozolino, L. (2014). *The neuroscience of human relationships: Attachment and the developing social brain*. WW Norton & Company.
Cozolino, L. (2017). *The neuroscience of psychotherapy: Healing the social brain* (3rd ed.). WW Norton & Company.
Crawford, A. (2014). "The trauma experienced by generations past having an effect in their descendants": Narrative and historical trauma among Inuit in Nunavut, Canada. *Transcultural Psychiatry, 51*(3), 339–369.
Crocq, M. A., & Crocq, L. (2000). From shell shock and war neurosis to post-traumatic stress disorder: A history of psychotraumatology. *Dialogues in Clinical Neuroscience, 2*(1), 47–55. https://doi.org/10.31887/DCNS.2000.2.1/macrocq
Culp, R. E., Watkins, R. V., Lawrence, H., Letts, D., Kelly, D. J., & Rice, M. L. (1991). Maltreated children's language and speech development: Abused, neglected, and abused and neglected. *First Language, 11*(33), 377–389.
Cunneen, C., & Libesman, T. (2000). Postcolonial trauma: The contemporary removal of indigenous children and young people from their families in Australia. *Australian Journal of Social Issues, 35*(2), 99–115.
Cunsolo Willox, A., & Ellis, N. R. (2018). Ecological grief as a mental health response to climate change-related loss. *Nature Climate Change, 8*(4), 275.
Danieli, Y. (1985). The treatment and prevention of long-term effects and intergenerational transmission of victimization: A lesson from Holocaust survivors and their children. In C. Figley (Ed.), *Trauma and its Wake* (pp. 295–313). Brunner/Mazel.
Davoine, F., & Gaudilliere, J. (2004). *History beyond trauma*. Other Press.
Duran, E., & Duran, B. (1995). *Native American postcolonial psychology*. New York Press.
Durkalec, A., Furgal, C., Skinner, M. W., & Sheldon, T. (2015). Climate change influences on environment as a determinant of Indigenous health: Relationships to place, sea ice, and health in an Inuit community. *Social Science & Medicine, 136-137*, 17–26. https://doi.org/10.1016/j.socscimed.2015.04.026
Dussault, R., Chartrand, P., Robinson, W., Erasmus, G., Meekison, J. P., & Sillett, M. (1996). *Report of the Royal Commission on Aboriginal Peoples*. Canadian Government.
Erikson, K. T. (1976). Loss of communality at Buffalo Creek. *The American Journal of Psychiatry, 133*(3), 302–305.

Evans, A., & Coccoma, P. (2014). *Trauma-informed care: How neuroscience influences practice*. Routledge.

Evans-Campbell, T. (2008). Historical trauma in American Indian/Native Alaska communities: A multilevel framework for exploring impacts on individuals, families, and communities. *Journal of Interpersonal Violence, 23*(3), 316–338.

Fast, E., & Collin-Vézina, D. (2019). Historical trauma, race-based trauma, and resilience of indigenous peoples: A literature review. *First Peoples Child & Family Review, 14*(1), 166–181.

Felitti, V. J., Anda, R. F., Nordenberg, D., Williamson, D. F., Spitz, A. M., Edwards, V., & Marks, J. S. (1998). Relationship of childhood abuse and household dysfunction to many of the leading causes of death in adults: The Adverse Childhood Experiences (ACE) Study. *American Journal of Preventive Medicine, 14*(4), 245–258.

Fleming, A. (2016). In what ways are indigenous Māori perspectives on attachment similar to and different from western psychoanalytic perspectives on attachment and what are the implications for the practice of psychotherapy in Aotearoa New Zealand? (Master of Psychotherapy), Auckland University of Technology, Auckland.

Ford, J. D. (2012). Indigenous health and climate change. *American Journal of Public Health, 102*(7), 1260–1266. Retrieved from https://ezproxy.scu.edu.au/login?url=https://search.ebscohost.com/login.aspx?direct=true&db=s3h&AN=77379313&site=ehost-live

Ganzel, B. L., Kim, P., Glover, G. H., & Temple, E. (2008). Resilience after 9/11: Multimodal neuroimaging evidence for stress-related change in the healthy adult brain. *NeuroImage, 40*(2), 788–795. https://doi.org/10.1016/j.neuroimage.2007.12.010

Gibson, K., Barnett, J., Haslam, N., & Kaplan, I. (2020). The mental health impacts of climate change: Findings from a Pacific Island Atoll Nation. *Journal of Anxiety Disorders, 73*. https://doi.org/10.1016/j.janxdis.2020.102237

Gone, J. P. (2013). Redressing First Nations historical trauma: Theorizing mechanisms for indigenous culture as mental health treatment. *Transcultural Psychiatry, 50*(5), 683–706.

Green, J. (2017). Radioactive waste and Australia's Aboriginal people. *Angelaki, 22*(3), 33–50. https://doi.org/10.1080/0969725X.2017.1387364

Griffiths, K., Coleman, C., Lee, V., & Madden, R. (2016). How colonisation determines social justice and Indigenous health—A review of the literature. *Journal of Population Research, 33*(1), 9–30.

Gundjehmi Aboriginal Corporation. (n.d.). *A history of duress - uranium mining on Mirarr land*. Retrieved from https://nuclear.foe.org.au/a-history-of-duress-uranium-mining-on-mirarr-land/

Halloran, M. (2004). Cultural maintenance and trauma in indigenous Australia. *Murdoch University Electronic Journal of Law, 11*(4), 1–31.

Hanlon, S. M. (2008). A non-Indian entity Is polluting Indian waters: Water your rights to the waters, and water ya gonna do about it. *Montana Law Review, 69*, 173–226.

Harlow, H. F., & Zimmermann, R. R. (1959). Affectional responses in the infant monkey. *Science, 130*(3373), 421–432.

Hartmann, I. C. (2019). Forms of expression of a preverbal reality in child psychotherapy. *Journal of Prenatal & Perinatal Psychology & Health, 33*(4), 259–281.

Hatala, A. R., Desjardins, M., & Bombay, A. (2015). Reframing narratives of Aboriginal health inequity: Exploring Cree Elder resilience and well-being in contexts of historical trauma. *Qualitative Health Research, 26*(14), 1911–1927.

Herman, J. L. (2015). *Trauma and recovery: The aftermath of violence–from domestic abuse to political terror*. Hachette UK.

Herring, S., Spangaro, J., Lauw, M., & McNamara, L. (2013). The intersection of trauma, racism, and cultural competence in effective work with Aboriginal people: Waiting for trust. *Australian Social Work, 66*(1), 104–117.

Hunter, E. (2009). 'Radical hope' and rain: Climate change and the mental health of Indigenous residents of Northern Australia. *Australasian Psychiatry, 17*(6), 445–452. https://doi.org/10.1080/10398560903062927

Jaakkola, J. J., Juntunen, S., & Näkkäläjärvi, K. (2018). The holistic effects of climate change on the culture, well-being, and health of the Saami, the only indigenous people in the European Union. *Current Environmental Health Reports, 5*(4), 401–417.

Johnson, D., Parsons, M., & Fisher, K. (2021). Engaging Indigenous perspectives on health, wellbeing and climate change. A new research agenda for holistic climate action in Aotearoa and beyond. *Local Environment, 26*(4), 477–503. https://doi.org/10.1080/13549839.2021.1901266

Kenney, D. (2012). Monumental failure: The Navajo tribe and radiotoxic wastes. *Hinckley Journal of Politics, 13*, 1–9.

Kinchela Boys' Home Aboriginal Corporation. (2017). *Kinchela boys' home - A conservation management plan: Unlocking the past to free the future*. Kinchela Boys' Home Aboriginal Corporation.

Kiraly, M., James, J., & Humphreys, C. (2015). 'It's a family responsibility': Family and cultural connection for Aboriginal children in kinship care. *Children Australia, 40*(1), 23–32. https://doi.org/10.1017/cha.2014.36

Krieg, A. (2009). The experience of collective trauma in Australian Indigenous communities. *Australasian Psychiatry, 17*(sup1), S28–S32. https://doi.org/10.1080/10398560902948621

Levine, P. A. (2010). *In an unspoken voice: How the body releases trauma and restores goodness*. North Atlantic Books.

Maier, S. F., & Seligman, M. E. (1976). Learned helplessness: Theory and evidence. *Journal of Experimental Psychology: General, 105*(1), 3–46.

Manso, J. M. M., García-Baamonde, M. E., Alonso, M. B., & Barona, E. G. (2010). Pragmatic language development and educational style in neglected children. *Children and Youth Services Review, 32*(7), 1028–1034.

Marsh, J. K., & Green, J. (2020). First nations rights and colonising practices by the nuclear industry: An Australian battleground for environmental justice. *The Extractive Industries and Society, 7*(3), 870–881.

Maxwell, K. (2014). Historicizing historical trauma theory: Troubling the trans-generational transmission paradigm. *Transcultural Psychiatry, 51*(3), 407–435. https://doi.org/10.1177/1363461514531317

McClellan, P., Atkinson, B., Coate, J., Fitzgerald, R., Milroy, H., & Murray, A. (2017). *Report of The Australian Royal Commission into Institutional Responses to Child Sexual Abuse*. Australian Government.

McGregor, R. (2002). 'Breed out the colour' or the importance of being white. *Australian Historical Studies, 33*(120), 286–302. https://doi.org/10.1080/10314610208596220

McNamara, K., & Westoby, R. (2011). Solastalgia and the gendered nature of climate change: An example from Erub Island, Torres Strait. *EcoHealth, 8*(2), 233–236. https://doi.org/10.1007/s10393-011-0698-6

Menzies, K. (2019). Understanding the Australian Aboriginal experience of collective, historical and intergenerational trauma. *International Social Work, 62*(6), 1522–1534.

Middleton, J., Cunsolo Willox, A., Jones-Bitton, A., Wright, C. J., & Harper, S. L. (2020). Indigenous mental health in a changing climate: A systematic scoping review of the global literature. *Environmental Research Letters, 15*(5), 053001.

Milroy, H. (2018). A call on practitioners to play a stronger role on intergenerational trauma. *Croakey*. Retrieved from https://croakey.org/a-call-on-practitioners-to-play-a-stronger-role-on-intergenerational-trauma/

Mohatt, N. V., Thompson, A. B., Thai, N. D., & Tebes, J. K. (2014). Historical trauma as public narrative: A conceptual review of how history impacts present-day health. *Social Science & Medicine, 106*, 128–136.

Necefer, L., Wong-Parodi, G., Jaramillo, P., & Small, M. J. (2015). Energy development and native Americans: Values and beliefs about energy from the Navajo Nation. *Energy Research & Social Science, 7*, 1–11.

Newell, P. (2005). Race, class and the global politics of environmental inequality. *Global Environmental Politics, 5*(3), 70–94.

Newton, B. (2019). Understanding child neglect in Aboriginal families and communities in the context of trauma. *Child & Family Social Work, 24*(2), 218–226.

O'Neill, L., Guenette, F., & Kitchenham, A. (2010). 'Am I safe here and do you like me?' Understanding complex trauma and attachment disruption in the classroom. *British Journal of Special Education, 37*(4), 190–197.

Paradies, Y. (2016). Colonisation, racism and indigenous health. *Journal of Population Research, 33*(1), 83–96.

Pearce, M., Eagle, L., Low, D., & Schurmann, A. (2015). Cut from 'country': The impact of climate change on the mental health of aboriginal pastoralists. *The Australasian Journal of Regional Studies, 21*(1).

Perry, B. D. (2002). Childhood experience and the expression of genetic potential: What childhood neglect tells us about nature and nurture. *Brain and Mind, 3*(1), 79–100.

Perry, B. D. (2008). Child maltreatment: A neurodevelopmental perspective on the role of trauma and neglect in psychpathology. In T. P. Beauchaine & S. P. Hinshaw (Eds.), *Child and Adolescent Psychopathology* (pp. 93–128). John Wiley & Sons Inc.

Petchkovsky, L., San Roque, C., Napaljarri Jurra, R., & Butler, S. (2004). Indigenous maps of subjectivity and attacks on linking: Forced separation and its psychiatric sequelae in Australia's Stolen Generation. *Australian e-Journal for the Advancement of Mental Health, 3*(3), 113–128.

Petheram, L., Zander, K. K., Campbell, B. M., High, C., & Stacey, N. (2010). 'Strange changes': Indigenous perspectives of climate change and adaptation in NE Arnhem Land (Australia). *Global Environmental Change, 20*(4), 681–692. https://doi.org/10.1016/j.gloenvcha.2010.05.002

Petheram, L., Stacey, N., & Fleming, A. H. (2015). Future sea changes: Indigenous women's preferences for adaptation to climate change on South Goulburn Island, Northern Territory (Australia). *Climate and Development, 7*(4), 339–352. https://doi.org/10.1080/17565529.2014.951019

Pocock, C. (2008). From segregation to assimilation: A thematic study of policies and practices Australia (1800 to 1970).

Pon, G. (2009). Cultural competency as new racism: An ontology of forgetting. *Journal of Progressive Human Services, 20*(1), 59–71.

Priest, K., King, S., Nungarrayi Brown, W., Nangala, I., & Nangala, M. (2007). Warrki Jarrinjaku Jintangkarmanu Purananjaku "Working together everyone and listening": Aboriginal child rearing in remote Central Australia. *Canadian Journal of Native Education, 30*, 61–74.

Ratnavale, D. (2007). *An understanding of Aboriginal experience in the context of collective trauma: A challenge for healing*. Paper presented at the Aboriginal and Torres Islander Mental Health Services of Central Northern Adelaide Health Service, Adelaide, SA, Australia. http://www.geocities.ws/pachsau/Ratnavale.htm

Redvers, N., Yellow Bird, M., Quinn, D., Yunkaporta, T., & Arabena, K. (2020). Molecular decolonization: An indigenous microcosm perspective of planetary health. *International Journal of Environmental Research and Public Health, 17*(12), 1–13. https://doi.org/10.3390/ijerph17124586

Reid, J., Taylor-Moore, K., & Varona, G. (2014). Towards a social-structural model for understanding current disparities in Maori health and well-being. *Journal of loss and trauma, 19*(6), 514–536.

Reynolds, H. (2013). *Forgotten war*. New South Publishing.

Rigby, C. W., Rosen, A., Berry, H. L., & Hart, C. R. (2011). 'If the land's sick, we're sick': The impact of prolonged drought on the social and emotional well-being of Aboriginal communities in rural New South Wales. *Australian Journal of Rural Health, 19*(5), 249–254. https://doi.org/10.1111/j.1440-1584.2011.01223.x

Rogan, M. T., Stäubli, U. V., & LeDoux, J. E. (1997). Fear conditioning induces associative long-term potentiation in the amygdala. *Nature, 390*(6660), 604–607.

Rothbaum, F., Weisz, J., Pott, M., Miyake, K., & Morelli, G. (2000). Attachment and culture: Security in the United States and Japan. *American Psychologist, 55*(10).

Ryan, F. (2011). Kanyininpa (Holding): A way of nurturing children in Aboriginal Australia. *Australian Social Work, 64*(2), 183–197.

Shriver, T. E., & Webb, G. R. (2009). Rethinking the scope of environmental injustice: Perceptions of health hazards in a rural Native American community exposed to carbon black. *Rural Sociology, 74*(2), 270–292. https://doi.org/10.1111/j.1549-0831.2009.tb00392.x

Smith, C. P., & Freyd, J. J. (2013). Dangerous safe havens: Institutional betrayal exacerbates sexual trauma. *Journal of Traumatic Stress, 26*(1), 119–124.

Smith, C. P., & Freyd, J. J. (2014). The courage to study what we wish did not exist. *Journal of Trauma & Dissociation, 15*(5), 521–526.

Sotres-Bayon, F., Cain, C. K., & LeDoux, J. E. (2006). Brain mechanisms of fear extinction: historical perspectives on the contribution of prefrontal cortex. *Biological Psychiatry, 60*(4), 329–336.

Stamoulis, C., Vanderwert, R. E., Zeanah, C. H., Fox, N. A., & Nelson, C. A. (2017). Neuronal networks in the developing brain are adversely modulated by early psychosocial neglect. *Journal of Neurophysiology, 118*(4), 2275–2288.

Stevens, B., & Bushell, V. (2000). The stolen generation: Psychological effects of the systematic removal of Indigenous children from their families and culture. *Ethos: Official Publication of the Law Society of the Australian Capital Territory, 178*, 17–20.

Terzon, E. (2015). *Darwin's Bagot community receives murals marking historical trauma of Indigenous residents*. Retrieved from https://www.abc.net.au/news/2015-09-25/bagot-community-gets-mural-makeover/6805590

Tilbury, C. (2009). The over-representation of indigenous children in the Australian child welfare system. *International Journal of Social Welfare, 18*(1), 57–64.

Tronick, E. (2009). *Still face experiment: Dr Edward Tronick*. Retrieved from https://www.youtube.com/watch?v=apzXGEbZht0&feature=youtu.be

Van der Kolk, B. (2014). *The body keeps the score: Mind, brain and body in the transformation of trauma*. Penguin UK.

Van der Kolk, B., Pynoos, R., Cicchetti, D., Cloitre, M., D'Andrea, W., Ford, J., & Teicher, M. (2009). *Proposal to include a developmental trauma disorder diagnosis for children and adolescents in DSM-V*. Unpublished manuscript. Verfügbar unter: http://www.cathymalchiodi.com/dtd_nctsn.pdf (Zugriff: 20.5. 2011).

Van Dijken, S. (1988). *John Bowlby: His early life: A biographical journey into the roots of attachment theory*. Free Association Books.

Vickery, J., & Hunter, L. M. (2016). Native Americans: Where in environmental justice research? *Society & Natural Resources, 29*(1), 36–52. https://doi.org/10.1080/08941920.2015.1045644

Waldram, J. B. (2014). Healing history? Aboriginal healing, historical trauma, and personal responsibility. *Transcultural Psychiatry, 51*(3), 370–386.

Walls, M. L., & Whitbeck, L. B. (2011). Distress among indigenous North Americans: Generalized and culturally relevant stressors. *Society and Mental Health, 1*(2), 124–136.

Walters, K. L., Mohammed, S. A., Evans-Campbell, T., Beltrán, R. E., Chae, D. H., & Duran, B. (2011). Bodies don't just tell stories, they tell histories. *Du Bois Review, 8*(1), 179–189.

Warin, M., Kowal, E., & Meloni, M. (2019). Indigenous Knowledge in a post-genomic landscape: The politics of epigenetic hope and reparation in Australia. *Science, Technology, & Human Values, 45*(1), 87–111. https://doi.org/10.1177/0162243919831077

Weir, K. (2014). The lasting impact of neglect. *Monitor on Psychology, 45*, 36–41. Retrieved from https://www.apa.org/monitor/2014/06/neglect. https://doi.org/10.1080/08941920.2015.1045644

Wensing, E. (2020). The destruction of Juukan Gorge: Lessons for planners and local governments. *Australian Planner, 56*(4), 241–248.

Whitbeck, L. B., Adams, G. W., Hoyt, D. R., & Chen, X. (2004). Conceptualizing and measuring historical trauma among American Indian People. *American Journal of Community Psychology, 33*(3), 119–130.

Wiebe, S. M. (2016). *Everyday Exposure: Indigenous Mobilization and Environmental Justice in Canada's Chemical Valley*. UBC Press.

Williams, J. (2012). The impact of climate change on indigenous people – the implications for the cultural, spiritual, economic and legal rights of indigenous people. *The International Journal of Human Rights, 16*(4), 648–688. https://doi.org/10.1080/13642987.2011.632135

Wilson, R. (1997). *Bringing them home: Report of the National Inquiry into the separation of Aboriginal and Torres Strait Islander children from their families*. Human Rights and Equal Opportunity Commission.

Yeo, S.-S. (2003). Bonding and attachment of Australian Aboriginal children. *Child Abuse Review, 12*, 292–304.

# 6

# Yarning About Racial Trauma

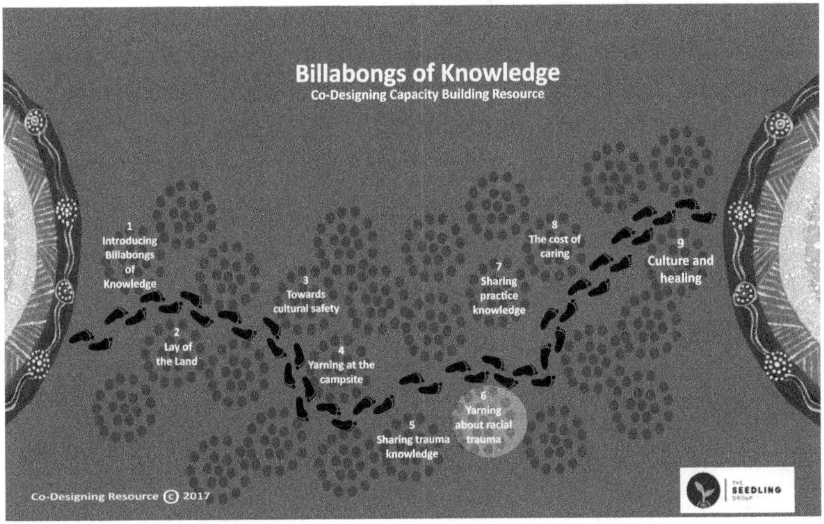


We acknowledge the traditional custodians of the lands on which we all meet today, from wherever you're reading this. We pay our respects to their Elders past, present and emerging. We thank them for the custodianship they've taken of all of our lands, holding our storylines and song lines and passing information down to our young ones.



N. Tujague, K. Ryan, *Cultural Safety in Trauma-Informed Practice from a First Nations Perspective*, https://doi.org/10.1007/978-3-031-13138-7_6

## Introduction

Racial trauma is a type of everyday trauma that has a huge and continuing impact on the social and emotional wellbeing of First Nations Peoples living in the colonised world. At this billabong we take the plunge and really talk about race, how racism stands in the way of the dignity and healing of First Nations Peoples. While it is challenging to talk about, understanding racism is also empowering. We discuss the historical and current policies that reflect the worldview of non-Indigenous culture and reinforce and continue everyday racism. We also cover the science of how racism makes us sick, impacting both our mental and physical health. We look at some of the different forms that racism can take, such as microaggressions, the differences between overt and covert racism and the seemingly innocent notion of a 'meritocracy'. We look at the 'cultural load' experienced by collective cultures and the chapter concludes with ways in which those who want to walk beside us, our allies, can contribute to the ongoing task of addressing racism.

**Activity 6.1 Five Senses Exercise and Check-In**

**Kelleigh**: Before you start reading this chapter, we invite you to go through this grounding activity with us. I took Nicole through the five senses exercise when we were in a recording studio for one of our webinars. First Nicole, tell me one thing you can smell.

**Nicole**: I can smell the smell of this studio I'm in. It's just a really clean, electronic lights sort of smell.

**Kelleigh**: Tell me something you can feel.

**Nicole:** I'm feeling a bit cold in my feet because it's the first day I haven't worn boots for a long time.

**Kelleigh:** Tell me something you can hear.

**Nicole:** I can hear a buzzing sound, a low whirring sound. Maybe it's the lights or maybe it's the air conditioning.

**Kelleigh**: Tell me what you can taste.

**Nicole**: I can taste the beautiful coffee I had this morning.

**Kelleigh**: Tell me what you can see.

**Nicole:** I can see the table next to me crowded with a whole heap of things. I feel really grounded now that I've tuned into all of that. Thanks, Kell.

**Kelleigh:** What's your checking-in word?

(*continued*)

**(continued)**

**Nicole:** I feel really weak in the legs today, a little bit wobbly. And that's probably a bit of tiredness and just excitement about this important topic.

**Kelleigh:** Give me one feeling word and where you feel it in your body, for how you're checking in today after doing the five senses.

**Nicole:** I feel calm, and I feel it all through my body.

If you've just gone through the five senses exercise, remember to think about the feeling word or emotion that's with you now. That's the last bit of pulling your body, your mind, and your heart together. This is a combination of a sensory motor and cognitive exercise.

## Notice Your Reactions

In Chap. 2 we spoke about how we make our worldview, how we build our knowledge system based on the information we receive from our caregivers and the world around us. We make rules about what knowledge we can accept or reject, based on the way we developed that knowledge system. At this billabong, we may talk about concepts and ideas which may challenge your existing worldview. If this happens and you have some kind of reaction, stop and just feel that feeling. Ask yourself: "why am I having that reaction? What worldview does this knowledge agree with or disagree with?" Sometimes the feeling or reaction might be in response to a history or forms of discrimination that you were not even aware of. In that case, the information may not be challenging your worldview but is consistent with it, and you may be reacting out of shock or surprise. Whatever lies behind your reaction, notice it and be aware that your body is responding and is trying to tell you something.

***Nicole**: For Aboriginal and Torres Strait Islander Peoples, learning this information for the first time can be a shock. When I first came across some of this research and Kelleigh and I started putting this information together, the feeling for me was of being validated. I now understood why I felt a certain way. It was a relief, but of course it was also a concern.*

Stay with us and keep an open mind before you decide whether or not you can or will incorporate this new knowledge while we yarn at this billabong. If the knowledge at this billabong leaves you thinking, "that doesn't sit right with me and I'm not sure how I feel about that", if possible, find a safe person who you can discuss the ideas with in more detail.

## What Is Racism?

We as First Nations Peoples know what racism is. We experience it every day. It hurts. It hurts to see it acted out against First Nations Peoples. That deep pain of racism is something that we have had to absorb and live with since colonisation. We know what it's like to have your money placed on the counter because somebody doesn't want to touch your hand; we know what it's like when our children aren't invited to the birthday party when everyone else in the class is. While it's almost invisible, it's a constant hurt that happens every day. Sometimes it's the hypervigilance you feel when you walk into a room. If something like a sticking plaster is skin-coloured, it's not *your* skin colour. You live in a world where who you are is not considered the norm. Because everything is normed to the dominant culture, *our* cultures, *our* identities, are 'invisibilised'. That's a result of racism.

How do we define racism? One straightforward definition from the Australian Human Rights Commission is: "*prejudice, discrimination or hatred directed at someone because of their skin colour, ethnicity or national origin, revealed through actions or attitudes*"[1] Not all racist responses are as obvious as this definition implies. Racism includes all the barriers that stop people from enjoying dignity and equity because of their race. It's important to distinguish equity from equality here. If you treat people as though everyone starts with equal privilege, you just reinforce existing inequalities.

Most non-Indigenous people in Australia would say they are not racist, yet we as Aboriginal and Torres Strait Islander Peoples experience it nearly every day. In annual surveys, about one in five Australians report having experienced racial discrimination during the previous 12 months

[1] https://humanrights.gov.au/our-work/race-discrimination/what-racism

(Markus, 2016, p. 60), and Aboriginal and Torres Strait Islander Peoples and certain migrant communities (such as African Australian communities) are much more likely to experience racism than other people (Markus, 2016, p. 67). In a survey taken in the years 2015–2016 (Blair et al., 2017), one third of respondents reported experiencing racism in the workplace. Research we and others did for the Queensland Mental Health Commission (2020) found that Aboriginal and Torres Strait Islander Peoples who were interviewed:

> demonstrated the general and pervasive nature of racism experienced throughout their lifetime and within diverse personal, family and community settings. Elder research participants considered that experiencing racism *'since they were born'* had complicated the ability of Aboriginal and Torres Strait Islander people to understand how racist behaviours impact their lives and wellbeing (Queensland Mental Health Commission, 2020, p. 4).

Everyday racism (Combs, 2018) is normalised; it's become the toxic water we swim in.

## Racism as a Fear Response

Racism has been described among other things as a fear response, a primitive survival mechanism, where one race unconsciously (and consciously) shows fear towards another race (DeSante & Smith, 2020). This could be fears for one's own level of security, importance or control. Remember that the threat response is a very primitive, primal one. It goes all the way back to when there was scarcity of resources, a scarcity of safety and food. It was quite understandable to fear not having enough, not being able to take care of your family. What happens is that people then create these exaggerated and negative beliefs to justify their reactions to people who are different from them in an attempt to secure their own safety and survival.

In Chap. 4, we talked about what happens in your body when you respond to threat. You respond from your base brain, the reptilian or survival brain, which activates your whole limbic system. This deactivates or minimises activation of your frontal lobes, your reasoning, problem-solving brain. On the one hand the person who's being racist is acting out of that primal fear; on the other hand, the person who's receiving that racism is also acting out of a primal fear because they feel under attack. This means we have two brains interacting from a threat response, each doing, saying and manipulating things to keep themselves safe.

That leaves each person with no choice but to defend themselves. Defending ourselves could sound like "but I didn't mean it like that…you're overreacting", which only shuts down any conversation about race, *leaving no room to learn*. Instead of trying to understand racism, we try to hold our ground, which becomes a lose-lose for both perpetrators and receivers of racism. To enter into a conversation where we can *learn*, we need to have our frontal lobes online. Everything else is reaction.

## Why We Don't Talk About Racism

One reason we find it hard to talk about racism in a constructive way is that we think about racism as all or nothing, you are either racist or not racist. We don't see it as a continuum (DiAngelo, 2018). We tend to think of racism like we do of pregnancy, you're either pregnant or you're not pregnant, you're either racist or you're not racist. If you do something that racist, you're automatically grouped in with the Ku Klux Klan. This is because there is a moral judgement attached to racism. If you're racist, you're evil. If you're not racist, you're 'good'. Thinking about racism that way shuts down any conversation. In fact, racism exists on a continuum.

It's important to recognise that there is a difference between being prejudiced, bigoted or discriminatory as an individual (you personally don't like or fear people who have black skin, for example) and being part of a society that has been built on racism, which is known as 'systemic' or 'structural' or 'institutionalised' racism Came et al., 2018; Durey et al., 2012). Racism is 'a system, rather than simply a slur. It is a prejudice *plus* power. It is designed to benefit and privilege whiteness by every economic and social measure' (DiAngelo, cited in Dune et al., 2021, p. 66). In this way, non-Indigenous people are the *beneficiaries* of systemic racism. We talked about this in relation to the idea of 'historical privilege' in Chap. 5

(Borell et al., 2018). No one who benefits from or has 'privilege' within the rules of that system can avoid unintentionally or unknowingly participating in racism. In Australia, systemic racism is so internalised, the system is so understood as the 'everyday predator' by many First Nations Peoples, that experiencing racism is one of the risks we as Aboriginal and Torres Strait Islander Peoples expect if we want to access the mainstream system.

To access Indigenous specific programs or services, the mainstream system demands proof of your identification as an Aboriginal or Torres Strait Islander person. To do that, you must be of Aboriginal or Torres Strait Islander descent, identify as an Aboriginal or Torres Strait Islander and be formally accepted with documentation by the community in which you live or previously lived.[2] This process is particularly difficult because of Australia's Stolen Generations, government removal from traditional lands, and loss of family connections due to the overrepresentation of Indigenous children within the foster care system.

Government policies were developed with the intention of 'breeding out' the 'Aboriginal race' (for example, *The Aborigines Act* 1905 in Western Australia[3]). Today, to identify as an Indigenous Australian, you are required to be 'spoken for' or endorsed by an incorporated Aboriginal organisation within an Aboriginal or Torres Strait Islander community. Importantly, identifying as Aboriginal or Torres Strait Islander is not based on skin colour. Ironically the burden of racism can also be heavy for fair-skinned Indigenous people because they are not protected by the black skin which might stop others putting their foot in it (Bennett, 2014). The burden of being a fair skinned Aboriginal person also has other consequences as expressed by this Aboriginal man from a remote community in Western Australia:

> As much as people say you're lucky you're fair skinned, you can fit into both worlds, I would actually prefer to be darker if I'm going to be honest

[2] https://aiatsis.gov.au/

[3] https://www.findandconnect.gov.au/guide/wa/WE00406

because it's more hurtful not being accepted by your own community than it is being called a black bastard by the white community (Oliver & Exell, 2020, p. 828).

We recommend having a look through the recent publication *Let's Talk Race* from the Australian Human Rights Commission[4] (2019), which is a guide on how to have conversations about racism in the Australian context. Another creative approach to talking about racism is the courageous conversation Aboriginal educator Daniels-Mayes (2019) has with her protagonist Master Racism, which we mention in Chap. 3.

## The Impact of Everyday Racism

Why is everyday racism so bad for you? Why does it have such horrendous outcomes? As a cumulative, ongoing trauma, everyday racism is like death by a thousand cuts. Those little attacks on you constantly put your system into arousal, filling your body with chemical, forcing you to make a choice, "do I engage in the fight or do I suppress my reaction? Do I run? What do I do?" It's like living in a constant battle.

### Everyday Racism Is Bad for Your Health

As racism is so common, we refer to it as an 'everyday trauma', meaning it is so prevalent and pervasive that it often goes unnamed or unchallenged, *but not unnoticed*. Again, we can analyse its impact by going back to the threat responses (befriend, fight, flight or freeze) we discussed in Chap. 4. We could say that not challenging everyday racism is an example of befriending.

***Nicole:*** *For example, I was visiting Cairns and my brother Chris picked me up from the airport. I had booked a room in a flash hotel and Chris and I walked into the foyer together. Chris has very dark skin, unlike me. As we*

[4] https://humanrights.gov.au/our-work/race-discrimination/publications/lets-talk-race-guide-how-conduct-conversations-about

*approached the young female receptionist, she smiled at me and then her eyes turned to Chris. There was a microsecond where her face froze and she didn't quite know what to say. Without missing a beat, he started joking and making light conversation. He was busy rescuing and befriending her without even realising it.*

For the perpetrators, it seems that we, the receivers of racism, don't have a problem with it if we don't challenge it. For the receivers, because we don't want to fight every battle, we inadvertently tend to the perpetrators needs, validate their beliefs and, in a way, befriend them. We can't possibly go to every argument we're invited to, but when we don't call it out, the everyday racial trauma continues to be reinforced.

When you experience racism as an everyday trauma, you may get a feeling you can't even name. What's happening in your body is you're leaving the Window of Tolerance and going into a threat response. The *sympathetic* part of your autonomic nervous system kicks in. Hormones like cortisol stream down into your body, getting it ready to react. But if you don't acknowledge it or do anything about it, you continue to soak up all of that stress hormone.

When the 'Black Lives Matter' protests were happening in America and around the world, including in Australia, some people carried signs saying, 'All Lives Matter'. If you are Aboriginal or Torres Strait Islander, you may have felt, "oh, that's so wrong". You just felt in your gut it was wrong; it's another manifestation of racism. Many people might have felt they had nothing to say in response to that, because on the surface, it seems logical, *of course* all lives matter. But the reality is that all lives are not treated equally.

What's happening here? When you read those signs, you felt something. Maybe you were unable to respond to that 'All Lives Matter' sign and were left in this invalidated and silenced space. That something was one of your worldviews being bumped up against. It was your fear response being activated, putting stress through your system.

That's why racism is bad for your health. It affects your heart. It affects your whole cardiovascular system. It causes high blood pressure, hypertension and heart disease. It affects your mental health (Ferdinand et al., 2013). Just like any trauma, prolonged exposure requires your brain to make some changes, both to its structure and capacity, as it continually works to determine what is threat or not threat. Racial trauma causes anger, distress, shame, depression, anxiety, isolation, which leads to other serious psychological and psychiatric disorders as well. It affects unborn babies, causes stress that contributes to low birth weights and premature births, which are prevalent in the Aboriginal and Torres Strait Islander community and other First Nations communities across the world (Brondolo et al., 2009; Harris et al., 2012; Hickey, 2015; Larson et al., 2007; McKenzie, 2003; Paradies, 2018; Mah et al., 2019; Ziersch et al., 2011).

## Everyday Racism Is Isolating

Everyday racism is isolating for individuals; it's isolating for communities and it creates stigma for whole suburbs and whole groups of people in community. Non-Indigenous people (often referred to as 'mainstream' by Aboriginal and Torres Strait Islander Peoples) may not be aware of how people in community feel about the way they are seen. We've had people in communities say to us, "mainstream looks at it as like this, they think we're all drunks, they think we waste our money". These communities were acutely conscious of those judgements; it was a big stress for them, how 'mainstream' sees their community. This is especially true if their community has been in the media a lot and only bad things are written about the people there. It's almost like people get too scared to say where they come from because they think they're going to be stereotyped and labelled because of how the media portrays them and the way they live.

## Everyday Racism Dehumanises and 'Others' You

We as Aboriginal and Torres Strait Islander Peoples understand that when you destroy someone else's culture, when you practise racism, you dehumanise the person. Once you start seeing people as lesser in morality, complexity or intelligence, you dehumanise them. This justifies setting up systems that continue to harm or control Aboriginal and Torres Strait Islander Peoples. When you think of ongoing racial trauma now, it's because *our mainstream systems continue to dehumanise us*. The onus of change then falls back on to the individual, but no one individual can change the system.

On a spiritual level racism threatens to erode your identity. It 'others' you. Othering is when you say or write things that put a gap between you and another group of people, you see them as 'not like me' or 'not like us'. For some First Nations Peoples, the act of othering challenges our sense of self belief and aims to tarnish our identity. Othering tries to convince us that we don't belong in our own country.

***Nicole****: When I'm marking my undergraduate student papers, I find myself often having to comment: "be very careful about using the words 'they, them, their' because as soon as you say those words, you're really saying, 'it's them, but it's not me'. You're putting that space between you and another group of people which makes them something different, lesser than you. When you make another group of people lesser than you, you dehumanise them, which allows you to do things to them you would not do to your own group."*

Many of us look back now at the failed Intervention in the Northern Territory in 2007, enacted based on allegations of child sexual abuse in communities and officially termed 'The Northern Territory Emergency Response' (Partridge, 2013; Vivian, 2010), and wonder "how could suspending Indigenous Peoples' human rights have happened in that way?" The Australian Government brought the army into communities. In order to enact the Intervention, the Government had to suspend the *Racial Discrimination Act* and go against the Constitution, which says that armed forces can't be used against our own people. To imagine it's okay to do that to a group of people, you would have to be a person who thinks: "well, they don't feel about things the same way I do, they wouldn't feel the same way I would if the army came into *my* suburb and took *my* children and tested *them* for sexually transmitted diseases. If that was in my suburb, that would be an outrage". The thought behind that is "they don't feel like that because they're not the same as us".

***Nicole****: That's the scary thing about othering. I always think about this when I hear about child removals, when babies are taken from Aboriginal mothers at the birth bed. I only have one son and I think: "if that happened, I don't even know what I would do, that is just unimaginable."*

Othering is also often unstated and covert, which means we don't always challenge it when we see it. The Northern Territory Intervention[5] was enabled and enacted through a combination of pathologising and dehumanising, with minimal questioning from the wider community. What enabled the Australian Government to activate the army to go in there was *pathologising* the 'other' and *weaponising* allegations of child sexual abuse. Child sexual abuse is a topic everyone in both mainstream and Aboriginal and Torres Strait Islander communities is concerned about, and investigating it is something that no 'good person' would actually question.

People don't like to talk about the Intervention. They don't like to talk about why they didn't say anything about it at the time, because it once again makes you think that you're either good or bad. It appears to imply some moral assessment of who you are as a person. A lot of people haven't even questioned what happened with the Intervention. Were people actually accused of sexual abuse? The Government was very public about enacting the Intervention but not so public about the results and repercussions.

## Everyday Racial Trauma: Racial Microaggressions

Colonisation disrupted everything for us as First Nations Peoples. It left us with a system that continues to enable and reinforce racism which impacts us on a daily basis. All those small acts of racism, called 'racial microaggressions', continue the racial trauma that colonisation unleashed.

This term 'racial microaggression' was first coined by psychiatrist Chester M. Pierce in 1974 (Pierce, 1974) to describe insults and dismissals he regularly witnessed white Americans inflicting on African Americans. More recently Derald Wing Sue et al. (2007, 2019) produced the most detailed and readable of papers on racial microaggressions, which we suggest you check out if you are interested both in the forms they can take and ways to respond or interrupt this type of insidious

[5] https://humanrights.gov.au/our-work/social-justice-report-2007-chapter-3-northern-territory-emergency-response-intervention

racism. Examples of papers that deal with racial microaggressions in Indigenous contexts include Hill et al. (2010); Houshmand et al. (2019) and Walls et al. (2015).

We discuss three types of microaggressions here: micro *assaults*, micro *insults* and micro *invalidations;* and share stories about our experiences with this form of racism. Microaggressions can be on a continuum from small interactions that are almost unnoticeable, to ones that are a bit more in your face, to more aggressive acts that are quite shocking.

## Micro Assaults

An example of a subtle micro assault might be, you're an Aboriginal or Torres Strait Islander person and you walk into a lift; someone tucks their handbag away in a nice safe place, or they grab their child's hand to make sure nothing's going to happen to their child. While it seems a very small act, it would still feel like a dagger wound to the Aboriginal person.

***Nicole****: I do remember this one day when Kelleigh and I were teenagers. We were on the bus coming home from school. Kelleigh was sitting on one side of the bus with her afro hairstyle and I was sitting on the other side. A non-Indigenous older woman got on the bus, looked around, obviously thinking, "where am I going to sit?" She went to sit down next to Kelleigh, pictured above with Mum and the huge afro she had as a teenager (Fig. 6.1). When this woman took a look at Kelleigh, something in her must have thought, "no, won't sit there," and she came over and sat next to me. We had a good laugh about that later. I said "Kell, she obviously doesn't realise that we're sisters and she just sat next to me by accident." Making a joke of things like that is what we do as Aboriginal and Torres and Strait Islander Peoples, because it helps to get rid of that stress hormone. It's funny, that was over 40 years ago and I still remember that incident. It's a micro trauma that changes the way you see the world forever.*

***Kelleigh****: Imagine what that message was to me as a teenager.*

***Nicole****: We did some research about racism and stigma in 2019 in a number of urban, rural and remote Aboriginal communities. A few guys from a large country town told us, "when three or four of us go to a shopping centre, we are asked at the door to split up and shop separately. We're not allowed to actually shop as a group". That was in 2019. I thought that was pretty in your face.*

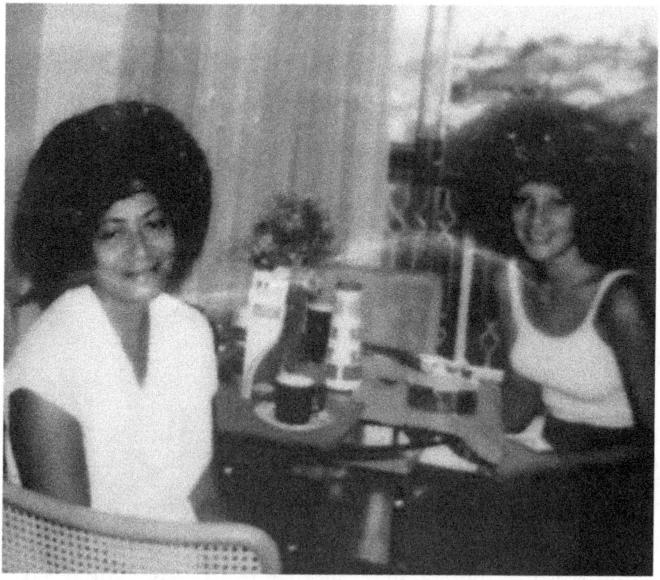

**Fig. 6.1** Kelleigh (right) with our Mum. Source: Family photo

***Kelleigh****: It was shocking to think that a human right could be so totally interrupted and that is accepted as normal. For the Aboriginal men to exercise their right to gather resources, they had to comply with such a discriminatory request.*

An example of a micro assault that is further along the continuum, one that's even more shocking and blatant, is the story of the Aboriginal grandmother who, when she gets into a taxi in Townsville, (and this is still commonplace there) is asked to pay her fare before the driver will take her to where she wants to go. The message is, "I don't actually trust you to pay your fare, so you better pay it upfront before we go anywhere".

## Micro Insults

Micro insults are small insults that may or may not be intentional; they could be just acts that are ignorant or insensitive. Sometimes it's hard to tell. At one end of the continuum, it might be something simple (but very common) like, "oh, you're Aboriginal. What percentage are you?" This is a very insulting question to ask an Aboriginal or Torres Strait Islander person. As a result of historical government policies, Aboriginal children were separated from their families and were judged according to the percentage of how much Aboriginality flowed in their veins (Bond et al., 2014). So-called 'half-caste' or 'mixed blood' Aboriginal and Torres Strait Islander children were considered more 'teachable' than 'full blood' children. They were the ones who were more likely to be taken away to live with white people or to live in children's homes and boarding schools (Wilson, 1997). Another intention of that policy was to 'breed out the Aboriginal' in the person. Ignorance about our history means that people who make these casual insults do not see them as insulting at all. Asking someone what percentage Aboriginal they are really just says, "I don't know anything about my history or your history, or the history of this country".

Another example of a micro insult is when a non-Indigenous person is looking for an Aboriginal person and says, "where's so and so? Has he gone walkabout?" Using the word 'walkabout' in that way is insulting because walkabout is a traditional cultural ritual (Yalmambirra, 2000). When people went on ceremony, such as for 'coming of age' or Sorry Business (a protocol when someone has died), walkabout was the respect of leaving the group or the community to go and pay their respects as part of that important business. It wasn't just about 'going missing'.

Possibly the most deeply hurtful insult for most Aboriginal and Torres Strait Islander Peoples is the ongoing celebration of 'Australia Day', the date of which marks the beginning of British colonisation of Aboriginal and Torres Strait Islander lands, as we talked about in Chap. 5. The fact that the land was taken by force and that sovereignty was never ceded, is still not recognised as the major insult it is to the First Nations Peoples of Australia. It's a difficult conversation to have because we all think of ourselves as Australians, Aboriginal and Torres Strait Islander Peoples as well as non-Indigenous peoples who live here and come from all parts of the world. To come up with a date where we can all celebrate Australia involves a lot of upset and anger on both sides. 'Australia Day' has recently become a day where white supremacist groups vocally make their presence felt in the celebrations.

## Micro Invalidations

The third type of microaggression, micro invalidations, is where your story or your lived reality is diminished. At the minor end of the continuum, it might be that non-Indigenous person on the bus who says, "why do you have to make this always about race? That's not racism. I chose that seat because I like to sit on the side that's not sunny." This diminishes what's actually happened from our viewpoint. Following that type of micro invalidation, what we do sometimes as Aboriginal and Torres Strait Islander Peoples is make little excuses for the perpetrator, which are called micro *validations*. So, if someone says: "why do you have to make it all about race?" I might say, "oh, she didn't mean any harm by that. That is just that generation." But you still feel the dagger, you still feel the wound; you still experience the threat response.

***Nicole***: *My experience of a micro invalidation that has stayed with me is when I went to a fashion parade with my girlfriend. A friend of hers came up to us and asked me something like "where do you work and what do you do?" During the conversation the whole story of the Stolen Generations came up. At the end of the fashion parade, when we were all having champagne and having a good time, she said to me about the kids who were stolen: "but they were better off, weren't they? A lot of them actually had a roof over their head and they had food and someone who loved them." That was very much more of an in-your-face micro invalidation and I felt I had to choose my words carefully. I said: "Actually that's not correct." I thought, "do I really want to get into this conversation about how wrong you are at the end of a fashion parade while I'm drinking champagne?" I made this little micro validation in my mind and said to myself, "she wasn't taught this stuff in school. She has no idea. She's just ignorant." But my making that micro validation doesn't take away the fact that my body went into hyper-arousal. I felt the injustice and the anger. I haven't forgotten it. It's burnt into my neural networks.*

***Kelleigh***: *And that person didn't learn anything new. She got to continue navigating her world thinking that her worldview was right. And that's such a harmful thing, not just for her, because she didn't learn anything, but for anyone else she runs into. It's important to remember that yes, while these micro invalidations make our history and our life experience invalid, our* *micro validations, that type of rescuing you got into with your friend's friend, is quite bad for us. If you think of coping behaviours like befriending as a threat response, then that micro validation is actually doing us harm.*

***Nicole***: *When I was at the fashion parade and I let my friend's friend off the hook, it was a type of freeze response. It felt like the accelerator and the brake were on at the same time, my body was just flooding with neurochemicals. And I was thinking at the same time, "I'm not going to mess up everybody's night tonight by making a fight out of this. I'm just going to let it go."*

***Kelleigh***: *The important bit there to remember is you were making yourself sick by having your system flood like that. I'm not inviting you to get into a fight every time. What I'm inviting you to do is be aware. Be aware that this validation stuff can make you sick and it doesn't change the conversation. And yes, it can be a tricky thing to manage.*

Another even more stark example of a micro invalidation can be how places are named in a way that reminds us of what happened in the past. Up on our Country there's a road called Murdering Creek Road, where a big massacre took place during the years of early colonisation (Gibbons, 2015; Williams, 2020). There have been lots of conversations in the area about whether to change that name to something less confronting. But the whole argument about changing the name is not because it was a massacre site and might offend Indigenous people, but because it's bad for real estate prices. This invalidates us as Aboriginal and Torres Strait Islander Peoples who might find it highly offensive, and we get that stab every time we see that sign. However, some local Aboriginal people feel that keeping the name is an important way of recognising the real history of that Country. We *could* validate it by saying, "well, they're right. It *is* going to affect real estate prices", but even knowing that's the reason behind the arguments invalidates and diminishes our lived experience.

## Common Themes of Microaggressions

Common themes that crop up with micro aggressions are stereotyping, exoticising and pathologising, all themes we buy into systemically as well as individually.

## Stereotyping

In 2014 a study was published showing that Australian media portrayed Aboriginal and Torres Strait Islander Peoples in an overwhelmingly negative light. The study of selected Australian media over a 12-month period showed that 75% of references to First Nations Peoples of Australia were associated with negative descriptors such as alcohol, child abuse, petrol sniffing, violence, suicide, deaths in custody and crime. Eleven percent of reporting could be considered neutral, while only 15% provided positive depictions of Indigenous Australians (Stoneham et al., 2014).

***Nicole:*** *A large percentage of my undergraduate students who are from other countries are met with beliefs like that when they come to Australia. They read about, see and often hear these beliefs from their fellow students. But when they start learning about the colonisation history of Australia, they're quite shocked when they hear what the real story is.*

That's an example of the power that stereotyping has. It's difficult for people who are the subject of those stereotypes, like the people we meet in communities who know perfectly well what non-Indigenous people think about them. It's that shadow we as Aboriginal and Torres Strait Islander Peoples live under all the time. Stereotyping dehumanises.

## Exoticising

This is where you glamorise a First Nations person's traits or culture, and make it look like a compliment. So as the receiver of the comment, you're not sure whether you're getting a compliment, or your culture is being made fun of.

***Nicole****: My experience of exoticising is with my hair, which is very curly. People would say things like: "oh, how many hours does it take to get your hair like that?" and "can I touch it?' It's annoying, I don't want people touching my hair or making a big thing about my hair. I'm not seen as a person first.*

***Kelleigh:*** *Or I get, "I love your brown skin, I bet you never get sunburnt." In fact, blackfellas do get burnt!*

Another form that exoticising can take is romanticising First Nations cultures. For example, Aboriginal peoples might be seen as more 'spiritual', or more 'cultural' than the non-Indigenous majority, which can be an objectifying stereotype. This quote comes from a nurse in Canada:

> I think my basic premise, especially with elderly Native people, is that they have a wisdom and a spirituality that many of us, I think, never achieve. They just know things (cited in Browne & Varcoe, 2006, p. 160).

This can be interpreted in more than one way. As the authors point out, the nurse's comments:

> could be interpreted as romanticizing or exoticizing First Nations culture … which has the potential to reinforce representations of Aboriginal peoples as exotic Others. At the same time, this nurse could be expressing genuine admiration for the elders she has encountered in her practice" (p. 161).

## Pathologising

The tendency to focus attention on Indigenous health issues prioritises symptoms more than what helps healing. We read and hear things about us, like how our lifespan is shorter, how we have more chronic illness, how we drink more, how we smoke more and so on. That becomes the story of you, and if you're not careful, you can buy into that story, but remember, that's not *our* story of us. That's a pathologising story that's put out there by others (Gorringe et al., 2010).

Pathologising has the power of othering, because it is the language used when the focus is on what is *wrong* with Aboriginal and Torres Strait Islander Peoples. It is the bias of mainstream science. When one worldview is privileged, everything is judged and measured by that. While this is an accurate statistic, a strengths-based view would ask 'what makes Aboriginal and Torres Strait Islander Peoples thrive and live healthy lives?' When we look at the strengths of a culture, we minimise our cultural bias. Fortunately, more recently researchers have started to look more at what's going *right* in communities, what's keeping people healthy, and the people who fund research are more aware of investing in that type of strengths-based research (see Chap. 9).

**Activity 6.2 Reflection**

What other examples of stereotyping, exoticising and pathologising could you add from your own experience of receiving, witnessing or unconsciously enacting these types of micro aggressions?

What was your first reaction when you read the Canadian nurse's statement about how she sees First Nations Elders? How did you see that response—genuine admiration or romanticising? What more would you need to know to support your view?

## Responses to Microaggressions

Identifying the type of microaggression you are dealing with can help you understand how or why you might respond. When it's a micro assault, the message is usually very clear, "I don't actually want you here. I don't want your kind here. I don't like this interaction we're having to have." With micro insults the meaning or intent is not usually so clear. They might make you question, "was that really an insult?" or "were they really that naïve?" Maybe the person is actually quite ignorant of the effect their words are having on the you. Once again, the intent or meaning is blurred, and we may be tempted to respond with a micro validation to keep the peace. There are some things that we as Aboriginal and Torres Strait Islander Peoples can do to interrupt the flow of racism and give us time to engage our thinking brains.

1. *Bring your frontal lobes online.* Instead of reacting out of that threat response, take a moment or two to calm your system, through a grounding exercise, such as a few deep breaths or a quiet self-hug, something to give yourself time to come back into the Window of Tolerance. Use your frontal cortex, your thinking brain, to assess the situation and ask yourself, "do I want to attend this fight and if so, what is it that I want to say about this?"
2. *Respond from your inquiring mind.* Ask a question that opens the conversation. Remember, the person who asks the question holds the power. While the other person answers, you have a bit of time to think about how you want to respond.

***Nicole***: *I like to say something like, "wow, is that really what you think?" That just gives me time because I'm clearly saying that's not what I think, but it's respecting the opinion that's been stated. It also gives me a moment to think about what I want to say next.*

3. *Use humour*. Humour is good to break up the intensity of the moment and move the energy out of your system. Our mob is good at humour. We use humour to stay in the Window of Tolerance, "wow, *really*? You think *that*?"
4. *Set a clear boundary*. This can be something as simple as saying, "it's not okay to ask me that."

***Nicole:*** *Now that I've had time to think about the situation at the fashion parade, even though it was a few years ago, if I had paused and had some time, I probably would have said, "That's not true. You need to go and find out more about what really happened."*

Check out Sue et al. (2019) for more examples of how to respond to microaggressions.

## Overt and Covert Racism

The original model from which we adapted this pyramid (Fig. 6.2) explains how overt and covert white supremacy functions in the United States. Our adaptation includes examples of common features of racism experienced by Aboriginal and Torres Strait Islander Peoples in Australia. It is divided into two parts: the top part of the pyramid (above the line) gives examples of *overt* racism that everyone recognises and that are not generally socially acceptable. Examples include racist jokes and racial attacks; things that policies and laws are written around; things we know are not okay; and things that 'weaponise' and make race the deficit, like calling an Aboriginal person who is drunk a 'black drunk', rather than just a drunk (you won't usually hear the term 'white drunk'). Another example of overt racism is the use of the term 'reverse racism' when an Indigenous person (or person of colour) is accused of racism against a non-Indigenous person. It is true that some Indigenous people can hold prejudicial views about non-Indigenous people as a group and act on

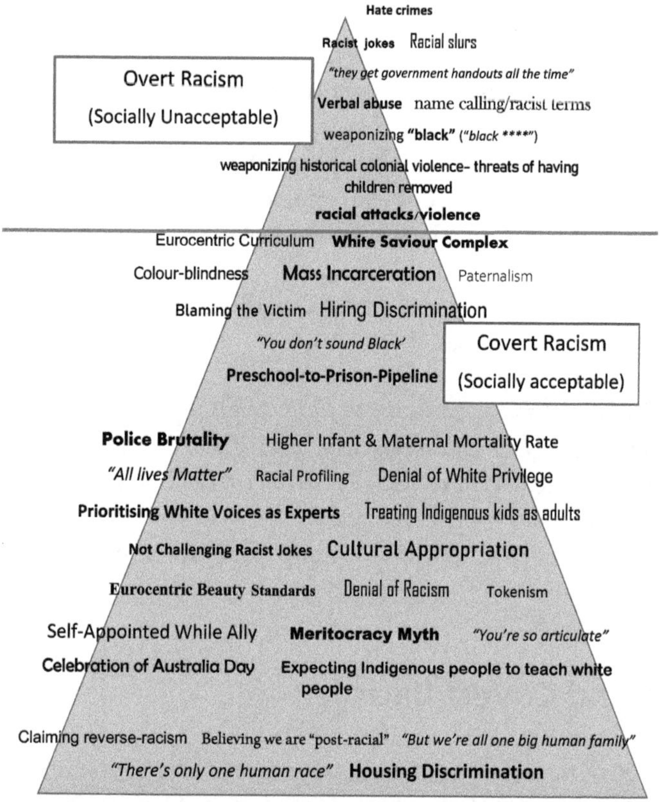


**Fig. 6.2** Overt and covert racism pyramid. Source: Adapted from *Safehouse Progressive Alliance for Nonviolence*, Boulder, Colorado, USA

those negative views. It does happen. But this form of discrimination or prejudice 'does not come with systemic privilege' (Dune et al., 2021, p. 66). The term, *reverse racism*, implies that racism should only be going in one direction, against Indigenous Peoples or people of colour. *Reverse racism* suggests that racism is going in the wrong direction, but aren't we just talking about *racism*? Accusing an Indigenous person of 'reverse racism' is another form of 'weaponising' race.

The bottom part of the pyramid (below the line) offers examples of *covert* racism, hidden racism that's more socially acceptable and often goes unnoticed or ignored, pretending it doesn't exist or doesn't count as racism (Kessaris, 2006). An example could be Australia Day celebrations, where even though every year there's been conversations and politics around changing the date, it's still socially acceptable to celebrate that day.

Tokenism is an interesting one. We know a story of an Aboriginal woman who was asked to be on the board of a company because the company was operating on contested land and making money from that unceded Aboriginal land. But that Aboriginal woman was never invited to any meetings. She wasn't consulted about anything to do with the company's actions. She only found out information about the company when she happened to get their newsletter because she was on their mailing list. The company could say, "we have an Aboriginal person on our board and we do get guidance around this". And yet the Aboriginal woman was never consulted. We call this being the 'token black fella'.

This is important, because every time you experience a microaggression, every time you experience racism, it hurts your spirit. There are many Aboriginal and Torres Strait Islander names to describe this sense of spirit that goes to the heart of who we are as First Nations Peoples.

If we look through the lens of this systems model we developed (Fig. 6.3), racism impacts us from a cellular level (when the body experiences a threat response), through to how we function as a global community (our systems and structures). Racism influences you as an individual, a whole human being, which influences your friends, your family, your extended family, your clan, your tribe, the group of people you belong to. That in turn influences the greater society where we all live in our own countries, which in turn influences the wider world.

We saw this connection very clearly with the Black Lives Matter protests in 2020–2021. What we saw happening on the streets in America affected us deeply as First Nations Peoples in Australia because it amplified how our legal systems tolerate overt and covert racism. How we make laws around what we do or don't do, how we care or don't care for each other and our planet, influences the planet itself.

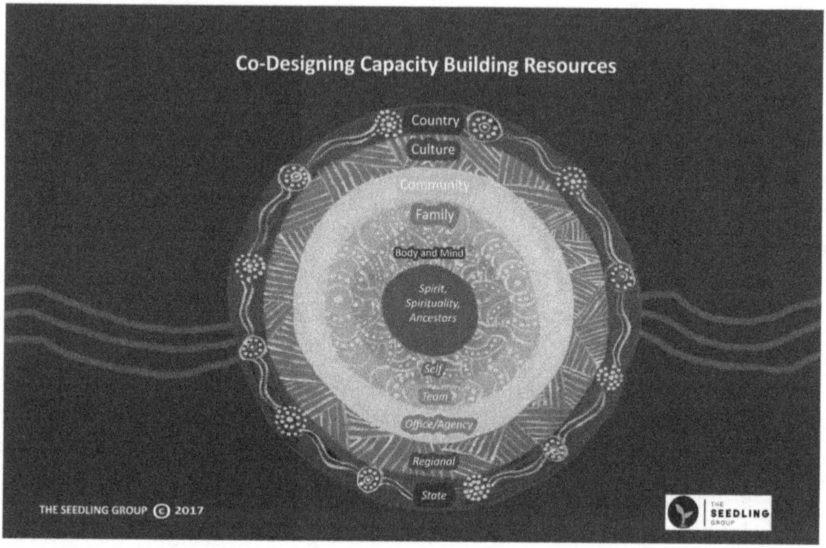


**Fig. 6.3** Indigenous connections: a systems model

## Meritocracy and Intergenerational Privilege

We're all brought up with that nice sounding idea of living in a 'meritocracy'. The dictionary definition of a meritocracy is 'a society governed by people selected according to merit'. There's a lot behind that word 'merit'. Who decides what counts as merit? If we go back to our discussions about the differences between non-Indigenous individualist cultures and First Nations collectivist cultures, the idea of merit certainly privileges 'success' as defined by individual achievements (Moore, 2012). Mainstream society encourages the idea that if you work hard, you'll be successful; you'll get a good job that'll make you lots of money and the harder you work, the better your life's going to be. That's the idea that we're all brought up with, that idea that 'good things happen to good people'.

The dark side of a meritocracy is if people deserve everything they get, then poor people must deserve what they get. If we praise rich people, then we have to despise poor people. They're not trying hard enough. If success is your responsibility, failure is your own fault. This idea completely disregards the privilege that some people are born into and it doesn't take into account systemic racism. If we buy into the idea of a meritocracy, we're buying into the politics of shame (Darlaston-Jones et al., 2014). This is a foreign individualist system imposed on a collectivist culture. Success in the mainstream system is measured in terms of money and credentials for an individual, which is at odds with what success means in a collectivist culture. Meritocracy privileges the Western idea of credentials; without them you don't have a voice in mainstream society. A meritocracy also doesn't recognise the realities of intergenerational or historical privilege, which we touched on in Chap. 5 (Borell et al., 2018).

***Nicole:*** *A good example of intergenerational privilege is when my son started university, he could come to me with his assignments and ask, "Mum, can you do a check on this for me? or "can you just make sure I've answered the question properly?" And I'd be able to say to him "you haven't referenced this properly," or "they're not going to like these references, go and find some more." That's a genuine privilege or advantage he has because I've been to university. If you're the first one in your family to go to university, you're on your own, basically. That first year of university is where you're just finding out about how to write an essay and what referencing is and how you should act and what happens if you miss an assignment deadline. If there's no one in your family to guide you through that complicated process, it will be more difficult for you to navigate the academic system. Remember that as late as the 1970s Aboriginal children could be denied access to education in schools in New South Wales. What I'm able to give my son is intergenerational privilege, which gives him every chance to succeed in a society based on a meritocracy.*

Another example of intergenerational privilege is access to inheritance. If you are white and middle class in Australia, you are more likely to receive some form of inheritance from your parents or grandparents. On some Indigenous communities where the law prevents you from having title to your traditional country, house and land ownership cannot be passed on in inheritances. Indigenous cultures are full and rich but don't subscribe to the meritocratic myth. As First Nations Peoples we have a different type of intergenerational privilege. This includes: the traditional privilege of connection and belonging; the privilege of family storylines and cultural identity; the privilege of the story of survival; the privilege of our grandparents' knowledge that they pass down to us; the privilege of knowing who our mob is.

Another form of intergenerational privilege is the notion of 'white privilege'. Have a look at the work by Robin DiAngelo (2011, 2018), a white American academic who deconstructs white privilege and what she calls 'white fragility'. This TED talk[6] of hers is thought provoking and may leave non-Indigenous readers feeling enlightened as well as uncomfortable or challenged. Keep in mind that she is referring to racism towards people of colour in the United States.

## Covert Racism Reinforced by Ongoing Colonisation

There is a long history of government policies in Australia that were designed to control Aboriginal and Torres Strait Islander populations since the beginning of colonisation (Fig. 6.4). Current policies are still influenced by the legacy of these historical approaches and ideas.

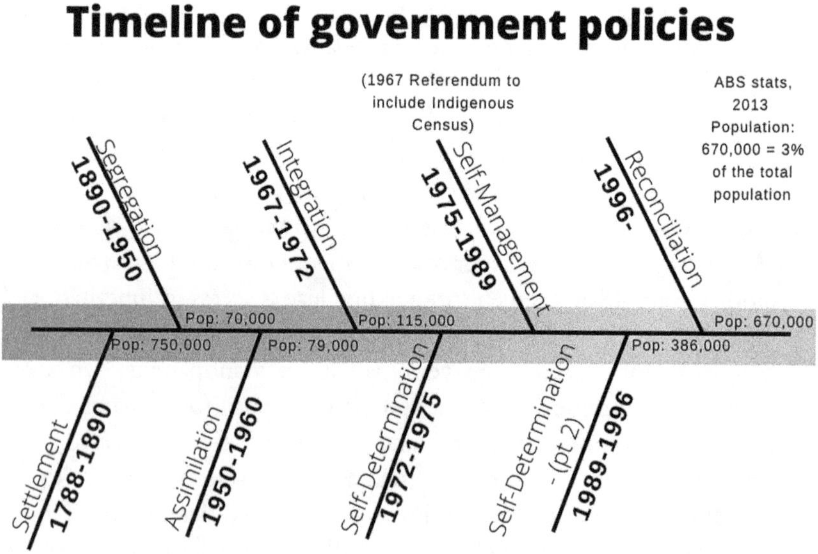


**Fig. 6.4** Timeline of government policies. Source: Developed from information in Pocock (2008)

[6] https://www.youtube.com/watch?v=h7mzj0cVL0Q&ab_channel=GeneralCommissiononReligionandRaceofTheUMC

This is a timeline that highlights the main approaches to government policy regarding Aboriginal and Torres Strait Islander Peoples from 'settlement' to 'reconciliation'. Each of those policies has dramatically impacted First Nations Peoples. As we mentioned in Chap. 5, it has been estimated that the Aboriginal and Torres Strait Islander population declined from about 750,000 in 1788 to 70,000 in 1950. That period was characterised by massacres and epidemics that decimated the Aboriginal and Torres Strait Islander Peoples. During that time people were rounded up and forcibly removed from their lands and ordered by government to live with clans they would never usually live with, clans with different lore, customs and languages (Pocock, 2008). It would be as unthinkable as removing people from different European countries to live together in one small space and expecting them to all get on, survive on a meagre imposed diet, and speak a common foreign language.

It is worth reading the report by Celmara Pocock (2008) that 'highlights the continuous process of colonial intervention in Aboriginal Peoples' lives, from the earliest colonial settlements to the present day' (p. 1). Despite all the attempts to deal with the so-called 'Aboriginal problem', from segregation to assimilation to reconciliation, we didn't go away. We are a resilient people. We're still here and we still have our culture that we're working hard to keep alive. It's important to recognise that current day policies are firmly rooted in historical racist policies and built on mainstream values that still don't work for us.

## Native Title, Land Rights and Stolen Generations

A good example of ongoing colonisation is the way Native Title and Land Rights are dealt with in Australia. This is a complex and fraught area of law, again reflecting the troubled legacy of government policies and attitudes since colonisation (see for example Strelein, 2005; McGrath, 2016). While some people use the terms interchangeably, there are significant legal and practical differences.

## Want to know more about Native Title and Land Rights?

**Native Title** law is a Commonwealth law, which means it applies to the whole country and is determined by the Federal Court of Australia. It came into law in 1993 after a landmark decision by the High Court of Australia the previous year, in which it overturned the fiction that Australia was an 'empty land' (*terra nullius*) at the time of colonisation (Borch, 2001). This was the now well-known 'Mabo' case (Hill, 1995; Chamarette, 2000), named after Torres Strait Island man Eddie Koiki Mabo who, together with other Torres Strait Island Elders, brought the case to the High Court (Hill, 1995). In brief, Native Title recognises the pre-existing and customary rights and interests that Aboriginal and Torres Strait Islander Peoples have on their lands. Claims can be made by representatives of traditional owners who need to prove they have maintained a continuous connection to the land.

**Land Rights** laws, on the other hand, are state laws, first introduced in the Northern Territory in 1976, much earlier than Native Title law. Land Rights claims can only be made by Aboriginal Land Councils on Crown land, that is, land owned by the state where the land is situated. The return of these lands is seen as compensation for dispossession and ongoing disadvantage for Aboriginal and Torres Strait Islander Peoples. There are restrictions on the type of Crown land that is eligible for a land rights claim, for example, land that is not being currently used; not needed for residential or other public purposes; and not subject to a Native Title claim. This means that if resources such as minerals are found on that land, those resources belong to the government or the private landholder. If a landholder is running cattle or sheep, they're still allowed to run their cattle and sheep. Land Rights claims are determined by the relevant state minister responsible for crown lands, not a court.

You see the bind, having Land Rights does not mean you have Native Title, and having Native Title does not give you Land Rights. If you are interested to learn more about the differences between Native Title and Land Rights in Australia, an easy place to start is https://www.creativespirits.info/aboriginalculture/land/land-rights-and-native-title-whats-the-difference.

This cartoon illustrates this bind we talk about above (Fig. 6.5):

The fact that you have to prove you've had *uninterrupted* connection to your Country in order to be granted Native Title is very difficult for members of the Stolen Generations in particular, where generations of people were taken from their families and their lands. Many who were taken as children don't even know what land they were taken from. They don't know which Nation they belong to.

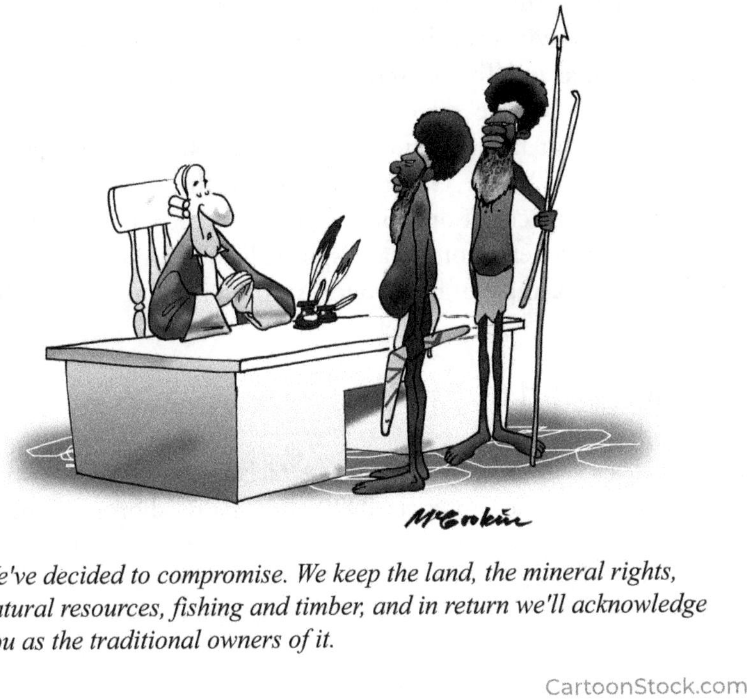


**Fig. 6.5** 'Native Title'. Source: CartoonStock.com

***Nicole**: We have heard many stories of people who have gone into pubs and someone has said, "I actually know you. You're related to such and such." And that's the first time they've learned anything about who they are.*

***Kelleigh**: Or someone comes up to them and says, "I'm actually your cousin," or, "I'm your brother or sister." And these people in their 50s have just discovered they have whole families they didn't know about. To finally find their families is so important and healing for members of The Stolen Generations. The organisation Link-up Australia continues to reconnect Stolen Generations people with their families and their lands, bringing them home, still bringing them home.*

According to The Healing Foundation website,[7] in 2018 there were 17,150 living survivors of the Stolen Generations in Australia and one in three Aboriginal and Torres Strait Islander people living today are themselves survivors or are directly related to a person from the Stolen Generations. Our family definitely is. We also know that one in seven people from the Stolen Generations lives with a profound disability, which has an impact not only on our social and health care systems, but also has an impact emotionally and spiritually on families and communities. This is an example of how policy is woven into our everyday lives.

## Cultural Load

Another legacy of systemic and covert racism is what is known as the 'cultural load' (Ketheesan et al., 2020) that many Aboriginal and Torres Strait Islander Peoples carry. Cultural load is the responsibility to live up to the cultural expectations we as Aboriginal and Torres Strait Islander Peoples have. This would not be problematic except that we are not working within our own cultural systems, but one that has been imposed on us. It forces us to choose between what our own culture tells us and what the non-Indigenous system requires of us. For example, caring for each other by meeting the obligations of our cultural protocols, such as attending to Sorry Business and engaging in other ceremonies that are healthy and connective, don't fit within the individualist system. This becomes a load because you have to choose between doing what is culturally right or do what the system requires of you. Many Aboriginal and Torres Strait Islander People give up their jobs when they have to go away for Sorry Business or have to care for their Elders. The non-Indigenous system is not set up to manage the amount of death and hardship Indigenous families deal with due to the huge disparities between Indigenous and non-Indigenous health outcomes, a product of ongoing systemic racism.

[7] www.healingfoundation.org.au

**Activity 6.2 Cultural Load Video (Fig. 6.6)**

We think the best illustration of what cultural load looks like for us is the way Aboriginal man Richard Frankland explains it in this video. [8] We have found time and again that the Aboriginal and Torres Strait Islander peoples in our training relate completely to what he says. It's both valuable and a good example of Aboriginal humour. Consider these questions during or after you watch this clip:

- What was different in the life of the non-Indigenous teenager and the Indigenous teenager?
- What other things would you add to the cultural load?
- How did you feel in your body when the cups were stacking up?

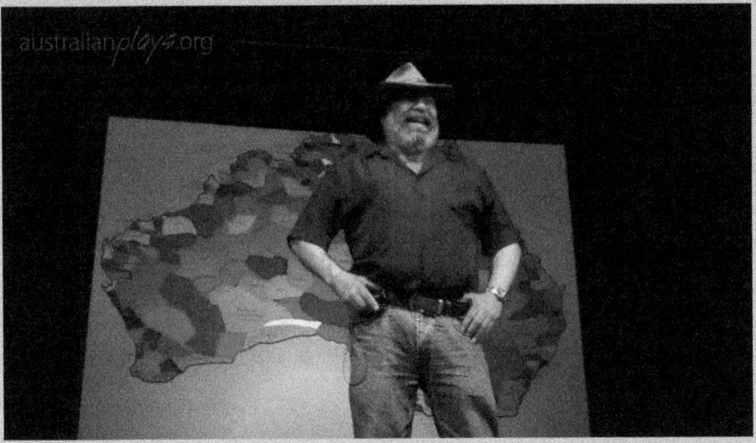


**Fig. 6.6** Richard Frankland Cultural Load Video (open access) with permission

***Kelleigh***: *I do love that Richard's a bit inappropriate at times and quite funny. The other thing I like about this video is that when he names the things that contribute to the cultural load we all carry as Aboriginal and Torres Strait Islander people, he is also talking about our cultural strengths. It just reinforces to me once again that our cultural strengths can cause trouble when they're married to a non-Indigenous system that doesn't acknowledge them and sees them as othering.*

[8] https://www.youtube.com/watch?v=E9AxZ2QseA0&ab_channel=AustralianPlays.org

***Nicole:*** *What I love about watching this clip with Aboriginal people in community is the way everybody gets sucked in and can really relate to what's going on in this young girl's life. I like how when he asks questions to the audience throughout, everyone gets into it. But we need to take the reality of this thing called cultural load very seriously and remember to self-care in a culturally safe way (see Chap. 8).*

## Tips for Allies

If you are non-Indigenous, it's not easy to be reminded of the realities of how it is for Indigenous people facing racism on a daily basis in a non-Indigenous society. Many of you may be wondering what you can do that makes a difference, how you can help, whether you want to be an active ally or know how to respond as a bystander when you witness racism (Nelson et al., 2010; Pedersen et al., 2011; Singh, 2019). If you are Indigenous and a non-Indigenous person has expressed the desire to be your ally and genuinely wants to work with you and be a support for you, here are a few basic tips that could be useful (also see Sue et al., 2019; Australian Human Rights Commission, 2019; Nakata, 2007):

1. *If you make a mistake as an ally, apologise, but not to the extent that the Indigenous person has to rescue you.* Don't go far into regret, like exclaiming "oh my God, I can't believe I did that" and keep apologising excessively to the extent that the Aboriginal person feels the need to come and save you or feels forced into a place of befriending or validating you. Be aware of how your excessive regret may feel for the other person, what might be going on for them. It can be another form of unaware racism.
2. *Don't expect an Indigenous person to speak for all Aboriginal and Torres Strait Islander nations.* This is very common, particularly for Aboriginal people in identified positions in non-Indigenous services or workplaces: everybody expects that person to be the expert on everything

Indigenous. There are hundreds of different nations, all with distinct cultural practices and lore. As Aboriginal people we are very conscious of these differences and know we don't have the right to talk for others or give you advice as a non-Aboriginal person on how to work with other peoples.

3. *Familiarise yourself with cultural protocols for Acknowledgement and Welcome to Country*. It is often the case that the only black person in the workplace or event is asked to do an Acknowledgment or a Welcome to Country. Firstly, if you are non-Indigenous or an Indigenous person who is not from that Country, it is inappropriate for you to do a Welcome to Country. It's important to understand that even when you are a Traditional Owner or descendant of that Country, you may not have the rights to do a Welcome, because of cultural protocols. It's important not to assume that an Aboriginal Elder or community member always has the authority to conduct the Welcome. You might say, "Are there any traditional custodians here who would like to do a Welcome, or would someone like to do an Acknowledgment?".[9] It is respectful to start any meeting or gathering with an Acknowledgment, even if there appears to be no Aboriginal and Torres Strait Islander Peoples present.

   ***Nicole**: Kelleigh and I come from Kabi Kabi country, but we've grown up most of our lives up near the Torres Strait and in Bamaga. When we do training on Kabi Kabi country, we don't do the Welcome to Country as it's not our place. We're still guests when we go on to our own country, as we don't have authority. Therefore we would do an Acknowledgement of Country.*

   The protocol is that whenever you are at an event or in a meeting, start with an Acknowledgment of Country, as we do at the beginning of each chapter. Anyone can do this, you don't have to be a First Nations person of Australia, but it's respectful and important for all Australians to acknowledge whose country they are on.

[9] For a detailed exploration of the complexities and 'controversies' around Welcome to Country ceremonies, see Bodkin-Andrews et al. (2016).

4. *Understand your privilege.* Understanding the privilege that a white skin gives you is not easy for everybody. We discussed the issues around white privilege earlier in this chapter and Robin DiAngelo's work is a great place to start to learn and understand what this means. You might also like to look at the work of Green and Sonn (2006), which looks at whiteness in the context of Australian efforts at reconciliation.

   ***Nicole:*** *I had a colleague at university who had a friend who used to say, "but I grew up in a foster home. I had a really hard life. We lived in poverty. My mum was a single mum. I just don't get this whole thing about me having privilege." And then she went on a trip overseas and she was in a country where everyone was black-skinned. When she walked into a burger shop the seas parted and she was served first. She later said to my friend "that's the first time I realised that my skin colour gave me privilege".*
5. *Learn about the real history of the Country you work or live on.* If you make a mistake and you realise you made a mistake because of your privilege or ignorance, don't expect the person you've just insulted to educate you. Go off and find out about the political and social history of the Country you're on, making sure your sources represent an Indigenous perspective. If you're going to work in community, the most fundamentally important thing you can do is understand the colonisation history of that community. Learn about what happened there and how that will inform how you work with the people who live on that community. There are many Aboriginal medical centres, agencies, land councils and their websites where you can get information.

## Concluding Comments

So why is it important to know all of this about racial trauma? Once we understand racism and its risks, we can embed protective factors into our policies. It's about taking you out of being fearful, out of that threat response mode. The risk and protective factors are similar for us all, whether we are a perpetrator, a receiver, a witness to, or a bystander of racism. Our practice is the product of constant reflection and refining. Take time to consider what we have yarned about at this billabong and weave it into your practice.

**Activity 6.3 Foot and Breath**

Talking about difficult topics like racism is normally quite anxiety arousing. So let's finish with the foot and breath exercise. Put your feet flat on the floor, either sitting or standing. Take a breath in and push your right foot firmly into the floor at the same time. On the breath out, release that foot from the floor. Just let the foot relax completely. Breathe in and this time push your left foot into the floor and release it on the breath out. Do that for three or four rounds, remembering to feel the pressure and the relaxation each time. This exercise is a sensory motor and cognitive activity.

**Activity 6.4 Check out and Reflection**

Now take a moment to check out. Do a scan of your body and sense how you're feeling and where you feel it after coming to the end of this challenging and provocative chapter. Then reflect on these questions:

- Note some experiences you have had that could be described as racial microaggressions;
- How did you respond to these?
- After reading this chapter, how might you respond to microaggressions or covert racism differently from now on?
- What difference could the learning from this chapter make to your family and community life?
- Note some examples of when you may have inadvertently or instinctively made negative assumptions towards a person because of their skin colour or cultural background.
- After reading this chapter, how might you respond differently in future?
- In what ways could you act as an ally to people who experience everyday racism?

## References and Further Reading

Australian Human Rights Commission. (2019). *Let's talk race: A guide on how to conduct a conversation about racism*. Australian Human Rights Commission. https://humanrights.gov.au/our-work/race-discrimination/publications/lets-talk-race-guide-how-conduct-conversations-about

Bennett, B. (2014). How do light-skinned Aboriginal Australians experience racism?: Implications for social work. *AlterNative: An International Journal of Indigenous Peoples, 10*(2), 180–192. https://doi.org/10.1177/117718011401000207

Blair, K., Dunn, K. M., Kamp, A., & Alam, O. (2017). *Challenging racism project 2015-16 national survey report.* Western Sydney University.

Bodkin-Andrews, G., Bodkin, A. F., Andrews, U. G., & Whittaker, A. (2016). Mudjil 'Dya' Djurali Dabuwa' Wurrata (How the White Waratah Became Red): D'harawal storytelling and Welcome to Country "controversies". *AlterNative: An International Journal of Indigenous Peoples, 12*(5), 480–497. https://doi.org/10.20507/AlterNative.2016.12.5.4

Bond, C., Brough, M., & Cox, L. (2014). Blood in our hearts or blood on our hands? The viscosity, vitality and validity of Aboriginal 'blood talk'. *International Journal of Critical Indigenous Studies, 7*(2), 1–14.

Borch, M. (2001). Rethinking the origins of terra nullius. *Australian Historical Studies, 32*(117), 222–239. https://doi.org/10.1080/10314610108596162

Borell, B., Moewaka Barnes, H., & McCreanor, T. (2018). Conceptualising historical privilege: The flip side of historical trauma, a brief examination. *AlterNative: An International Journal of Indigenous Peoples, 14*(1), 25–34.

Brondolo, E., Brady ver Halen, N., Pencille, M., Beatty, D., & Contrada, R. J. (2009). Coping with racism: A selective review of the literature and a theoretical and methodological critique. *Journal of Behavioral Medicine, 32*(1), 64–88. https://doi.org/10.1007/s10865-008-9193-0

Browne, A. J., & Varcoe, C. (2006). Critical cultural perspectives and health care involving Aboriginal peoples. *Contemporary nurse, 22*(2), 155–168.

Came, H., Doole, C., McKenna, B., & McCreanor, T. (2018). Institutional racism in public health contracting: Findings of a nationwide survey from New Zealand. *Social Science & Medicine, 199*, 132–139. https://doi.org/10.1016/j.socscimed.2017.06.002

Chamarette, C. (2000). Terra Nullius then and now: Mabo, Native Title, and reconciliation in 2000. *Australian Psychologist, 35*(2), 167–172. https://doi.org/10.1080/00050060008260339

Combs, B. H. (2018). Everyday racism is still racism: The role of place in theorizing continuing racism in modern US society. *Phylon, 55*(1 & 2), 38–59.

Daniels-Mayes, S. (2019). A courageous conversation with racism: Revealing the racialised stories of Aboriginal deficit for pre-service teachers. *The Australian Educational Researcher, 47*, 537–554. https://doi.org/10.1007/s13384-019-00360-0

Darlaston-Jones, D., Herbert, J., Ryan, K., Darlaston-Jones, W., Harris, J., & Dudgeon, P. (2014). Are we asking the right questions? Why we should have a decolonzing discourse based on conscientization rather than indigenizing the curriculum. *Canadian Journal of Native Education, 37*(1), 86–104.

DeSante, C. D., & Smith, C. W. (2020). Fear, institutionalized racism, and empathy: The underlying dimensions of whites' racial attitudes. *PS. Political Science & Politics, 53*(4), 639–645. https://doi.org/10.1017/S1049096520000414

DiAngelo, R. (2010). Why can't we all just be individuals?: Countering the discourse of individualism in anti-racist education. *InterActions: UCLA Journal of Education and Information Studies, 6*(1), 1–25. Retrieved from https://escholarship.org/uc/item/5fm4h8wm

DiAngelo, R. (2011). White fragility. *International Journal of Critical Pedagogy, 3*(3), 54–70.

DiAngelo, R. (2018). *White fragility: Why it's so hard for white people to talk about racism*. Beacon Press.

Dune, T., McLeod, K., & Williams, R. (Eds.). (2021). *Culture, diversity and health in Australia: Towards culturally safe health care*. Routledge.

Durey, A., Thompson, S. C., & Wood, M. (2012). Time to bring down the twin towers in poor Aboriginal hospital care: Addressing institutional racism and misunderstandings in communication. *Internal Medicine Journal, 42*(1), 17–22. https://doi.org/10.1111/j.1445-5994.2011.02628.x

Ferdinand, A., Paradies, Y., & Kelaher, M. (2013). *Mental health impacts of racial discrimination in Victorian Aboriginal communities: The localities embracing and accepting diversity (LEAD) experiences of racism survey*. The Lowitja Institute.

Gibbons, R. (2015). *Deconstructing colonial myths: The myth of murdering creek*. (Self-published), Academia.

Gorringe, S. D., Ross, J., & Fforde, C. (2010). *'Will the real Aborigine please stand up': Strategies for breaking the stereotypes and changing the conversation*. Australian Institute of Aboriginal and Torres Strait Islander Studies.

Green, M. J., & Sonn, C. C. (2006). Problematising the discourses of the dominant: Whiteness and reconciliation. *Journal of Community & Applied Social Psychology, 16*(5), 379–395. https://doi.org/10.1002/casp.882

Harris, R., Cormack, D., Tobias, M., Yeh, L.-C., Talamaivao, N., Minster, J., & Timutimu, R. (2012). The pervasive effects of racism: Experiences of racial discrimination in New Zealand over time and associations with multiple health domains. *Social Science & Medicine, 74*(3), 408–415. https://doi.org/10.1016/j.socscimed.2011.11.004

Hickey, S. D. (2015). 'They say I'm not a typical Blackfella': Experiences of racism and ontological insecurity in urban Australia. *Journal of Sociology, 52*(4), 725–740. https://doi.org/10.1177/1440783315581218

Hill, R. P. (1995). Blackfellas and whitefellas: Aboriginal land rights, the Mabo decision, and the meaning of land. *Human Rights Quarterly, 17*(2), 303–322.

Hill, J. S., Kim, S., & Williams, C. D. (2010). The context of racial microaggressions against indigenous peoples. In D. W. Sue (Ed.), *Microaggressions and marginality: Manifestation, dynamics, and impact* (pp. 105–122). John Wiley & Sons.

Houshmand, S., Spanierman, L. B., & De Stefano, J. (2019). "I have strong medicine, you see": Strategic responses to racial microaggressions. *Journal of Counseling Psychology, 66*(6), 651–664.

Kessaris, T. N. (2006). About being Mununga (Whitefulla): Making covert group racism visible. *Journal of Community & Applied Social Psychology, 16*(5), 347–362. https://doi.org/10.1002/casp.880

Ketheesan, S., Rinaudo, M., Berger, M., Wenitong, M., Juster, R. P., McEwen, B. S., & Sarnyai, Z. (2020). Stress, allostatic load and mental health in Indigenous Australians. *Stress, 23*(5), 509–518. https://doi.org/10.1080/10253890.2020.1732346

Larson, A., Gillies, M., Howard, P. J., & Coffin, J. (2007). It's enough to make you sick: the impact of racism on the health of Aboriginal Australians. *Australian and New Zealand Journal of Public Health, 31*(4), 322–329. https://doi.org/10.1111/j.1753-6405.2007.00079.x

Mah, B. L., Pringle, K. G., Weatherall, L., Keogh, L., Schumacher, T., Eades, S., Brown, A., Lumbers, E. R., Roberts, C. T., Diehm, C., Smith, R., & Rae, K. M. (2019). Pregnancy stress, healthy pregnancy and birth outcomes – The need for early preventative approaches in pregnant Australian Indigenous women: A prospective longitudinal cohort study. *Journal of Developmental Origins of Health and Disease, 10*(1), 31–38. https://doi.org/10.1017/S204017441800079X

Markus, A. B. (2016). *Australians today: The Australia@ 2015 Scanlon foundation survey*. Australian Centre for Jewish Civilisation Monash University.

McGrath, P. (Ed.). (2016). *The right to protect sites: Indigenous heritage management in the era of Native Title*. Australian Institute of Aboriginal and Torres Strait Islander Studies.

McKenzie, K. (2003). Racism and health. *BMJ: British Medical Journal, 326*(7380), 65. https://doi.org/10.1136/bmj.326.7380.65

Moore, R. (2012). Whitewashing the gap: The discursive practices of whiteness. *International Journal of Critical Indigenous Studies, 5*(2), 2–12.

Nakata, M. N. (2007). *Disciplining the savages, savaging the disciplines.* Aboriginal Studies Press.

Nelson, J., Dunn, K. M., Paradies, Y., Pedersen, A., Sharpe, S., Hynes, M., & Guerin, B. (2010). *Review of Bystander approaches in support of preventing race-based discrimination (1921822058).* Victorian Health Promotion Foundation.

Oliver, R., & Exell, M. (2020). Identity, translanguaging, linguicism and racism: The experience of Australian Aboriginal people living in a remote community. *International Journal of Bilingual Education and Bilingualism, 23*(7), 819–832.

Paradies, Y. (2018). Racism and indigenous health. *Oxford Research Encyclopedia of Global Public Health.* Retrieved from https://oxfordre.com/publichealth/view/10.1093/acrefore/9780190632366.001.0001/acrefore-9780190632366-e-86. https://doi.org/10.1093/acrefore/9780190632366.013.86

Partridge, E. (2013). Caught in the same frame? The language of evidence-based policy in debates about the Australian Government 'Intervention' into Northern Territory Aboriginal Communities. *Social Policy & Administration, 47*(4), 399–415. https://doi.org/10.1111/spol.12026

Pedersen, A., Paradies, Y., Hartley, L. K., & Dunn, K. M. (2011). Bystander antiprejudice: Cross-cultural education, links with positivity towards cultural 'outgroups' and preparedness to speak out. *Journal of Pacific Rim Psychology, 5*(1), 19–30.

Pierce, C. M. (1974). Psychiatric problems of the Black minority. In S. Arietti (Ed.), *American Handbook of Psychiatry* (pp. 512–523). Basic Books.

Pocock, C. (2008). *'From segregation to assimilation': A thematic study of policies and practices in Australia 1800 – 1970.* The University of Queensland.

Queensland Mental Health Commission. (2020). *Don't judge, and listen: Experiences of stigma and discrimination related to problematic alcohol and other drug use.* Retrieved from https://www.qmhc.qld.gov.au/sites/default/files/qmhc_dont_judge_and_listen_report.pdf

Singh, A. A. (2019). *The racial healing handbook: Practical activities to help you challenge privilege, confront systemic racism, and engage in collective healing.* New Harbinger Publications.

Stoneham, M., Goodman, J., & Daube, M. (2014). The portrayal of indigenous health in selected Australian media. *The International Indigenous Policy Journal, 5*(1), 1–13.

Strelein, L. (2005). From Mabo to Yorta Yorta: Native Title law in Australia. *Washington University Journal of Law and Policy, 19*, 225–271.

Sue, D. W., Capodilupo, C. M., Torino, G. C., Bucceri, J. M., Holder, A., Nadal, K. L., & Esquilin, M. (2007). Racial microaggressions in everyday life: Implications for clinical practice. *American Psychologist, 62*(4), 271.

Sue, D. W., Alsaidi, S., Awad, M. N., Glaeser, E., Calle, C. Z., & Mendez, N. (2019). Disarming racial microaggressions: Microintervention strategies for targets, White allies, and bystanders. *American Psychologist, 74*(1), 128–142.

Vivian, A. (2010). Some human rights are worth more than others: The Northern Territory Intervention and the Alice Springs Town Camps. *Alternative Law Journal, 35*(1), 13–17. https://doi.org/10.1177/1037969X1003500103

Walls, M. L., Gonzalez, J., Gladney, T., & Onello, E. (2015). Unconscious biases: Racial microaggressions in American Indian health care. *The Journal of the American Board of Family Medicine, 28*(2), 231–239.

Williams, P. A. (2020). Murdering creek. *Chicago Quarterly Review, 30*(The Australian Issue), 259–264.

Wilson, R. (1997). *Bringing Them Home: Report of the national inquiry into the separation of Aboriginal and Torres Strait Islander children from their families.* Human Rights and Equal Opportunity Commission.

Yalmambirra. (2000). Black time… white time: My time… your time. *Journal of Occupational Science, 7*(3), 133–137.

Ziersch, A. M., Gallaher, G., Baum, F., & Bentley, M. (2011). Responding to racism: Insights on how racism can damage health from an urban study of Australian Aboriginal people. *Social Science & Medicine, 73*(7), 1045–1053. https://doi.org/10.1016/j.socscimed.2011.06.058

# 7

# Sharing Practice Knowledge: Trauma-Informed Practice

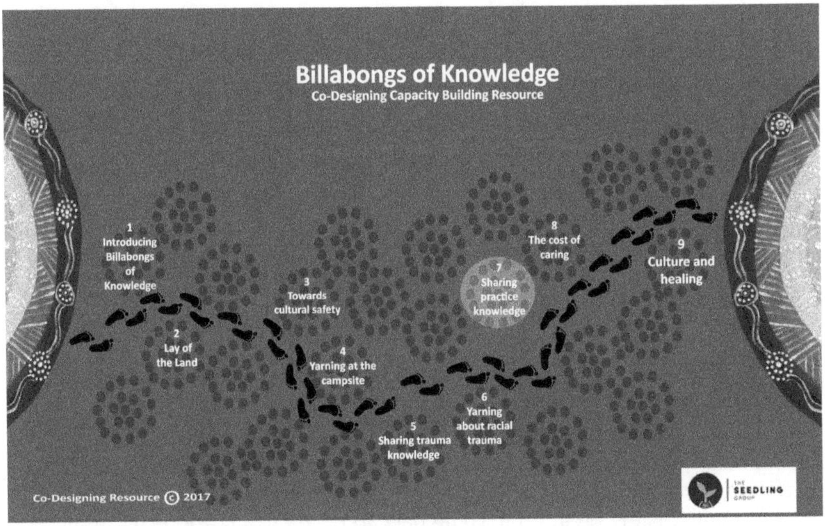


We pay our respects to the peoples whose lands we are gathered on today. We acknowledge Elders, past, present and emerging. We also acknowledge the wonderful custodianship of the land that we are on and look forward to playing our part in that custodianship.


N. Tujague, K. Ryan, *Cultural Safety in Trauma-Informed Practice from a First Nations Perspective*, https://doi.org/10.1007/978-3-031-13138-7_7

## Introduction

This billabong is all about sharing practice knowledge. Specifically, we share knowledge about cultural safety in trauma-informed practice. What does that actually mean? We have knowledge based on neuroscience that complements Indigenous Knowledge practices and provides validation for the western system. Western science now allows us to map and show what's happening in the brain and the body when we do healing work with our clients and communities. Although we know that psychological trauma is very prevalent in our societies, as practitioners we still can't always know who has a trauma story and who hasn't. Many people don't even know their own trauma stories. If we work in a trauma-informed and culturally safe way, we provide an environment that does no harm and also promotes holistic healing that is consistent with First Nations values and practices. At this billabong we revisit the Social and Emotional Wellbeing Wheel and the Circle of Knowledge models as frameworks for decolonising practice and working in a *culturally safe way*. We go on to unpack principles and models that are essential for working in a *trauma-informed way*, including evidence-based strategies that deal with collective trauma, as well as individual trauma.

**Activity 7.1 Grounding Exercise**

Stand with your feet just under your hips, not wide apart; just nice and central and balanced. Put your hands loosely by your side. Take a breath in and lean as far forward as you can without falling over. Hold. Really feel the strain on your body. On the breath out, come back to centre. Do that one more time, breathe in, come forward; breathe out, come back to centre. On the next breath in, move to your right, keeping your left foot on the ground, lean as far as you can without falling. Hold. Breathe out, come back to centre. Repeat one more time. Breathe in, move to your left, keeping your right foot on the ground. Hold. Breathe out, back to centre. Repeat one more time. Now just give your body a bit of a shake, shake it out. Your body should now be awake and present. This is an example of a cognitive, sensory-motor exercise.

**Activity 7.2 Check in**

Take a moment to tune into your body, think about what you can feel in your body, and connect that feeling to your thoughts and give it a feeling word.

## Decolonising Practice: The Social and Emotional Wellbeing Wheel

As our focus is on what is important about trauma-informed practice with Aboriginal and Torres Strait Islander Peoples, it becomes apparent that there are two very different worldviews at play. If you only privilege your own worldview, you could hinder your client's recovery and wellbeing by missing critical elements necessary for their healing. As we talk about in Chap. 2, the Social and Emotional Wellbeing Wheel (Fig. 7.1)

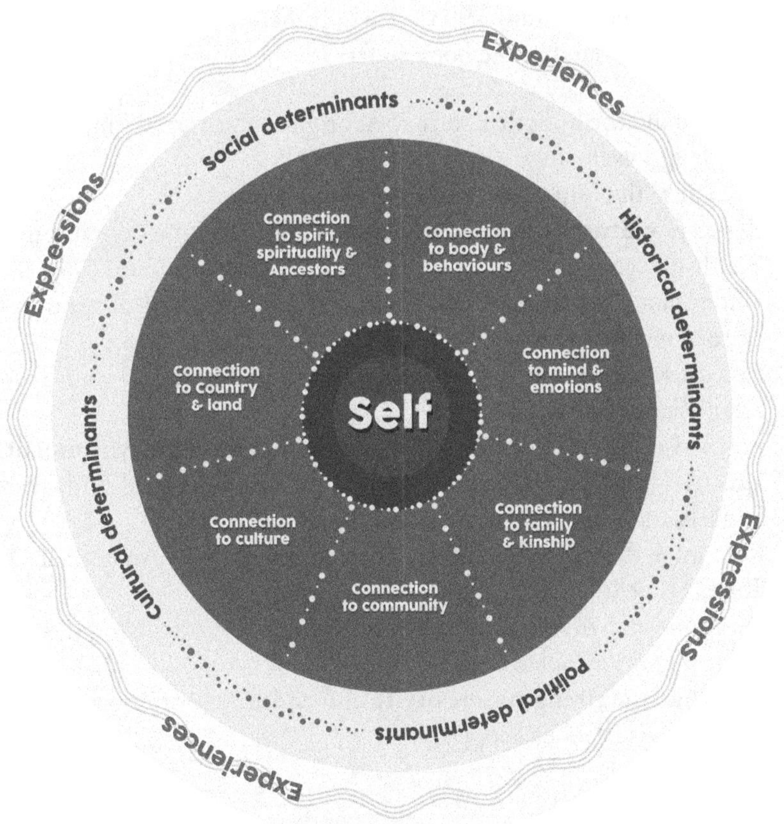


Fig. 7.1 Social and Emotional Wellbeing Wheel

shows that it's not all about symptoms and pathology for Aboriginal and Torres Strait Islander Peoples. Our wellbeing is as much about our connection to land and our connection to kinship as it is about what our individual symptoms are.

As we also mention in Chap. 2, if you're working with Aboriginal and Torres Strait Islander clients, or you're working in your community, have the Social and Emotional Wellbeing Wheel available for you and your client to check in with on a regular basis. If you are a non-Indigenous worker, this will help create trust and cultural safety for your Indigenous clients.

The Wheel is based on nine principles, drawn from the 'Ways Forward' Report (Raphael & Swan, 1995). These principles summarise much of what we have covered in the book so far:

1. Understand the **holistic** nature of Aboriginal and Torres Strait Islander health and wellbeing;
2. Recognise the centrality of **self-determination;**
3. Respect **culturally valid understandings** in the provision of health services;
4. Understand that **trauma and loss** are a direct result of disruption to cultural wellbeing;
5. Recognise and respect the **human rights** of Aboriginal and Torres Strait Islander Peoples;
6. Recognise the negative impact that **racism, stigma, environmental adversity and social disadvantage** have on Aboriginal and Torres Strait Islander mental health and wellbeing;
7. Recognise the centrality of **family and kinship** to Aboriginal and Torres Strait Islander Peoples;
8. Recognise the **diversity of ways of living** of Aboriginal and Torres Strait Islander Peoples;
9. Recognise the **strengths, creativity and endurance** of Aboriginal and Torres Strait Islander Peoples.[1]

---

[1] For more information on the SEWB Wheel see https://timhwb.org.au/fact-sheets/

You can read more about examples of the Social and Emotional Wellbeing Wheel in practice in Chap. 2.

## Decolonising Practice: Circles of Knowledge and Connection

In Chap. 4 we introduce you to the Circles of Knowledge and Connection (Fig. 7.2), another model that maps connection to country, language, ancestors and kinship, to mental and physical wellbeing. It is a representation of the long history of wellbeing and healing knowledge in First Nations cultures. A poster of the Circle of Knowledge model could also be something you could have on hand to refer to and ask yourself, "how can I extend my clinical understanding in a way that aligns more with First Nations cultural values and restores cultural healing?"

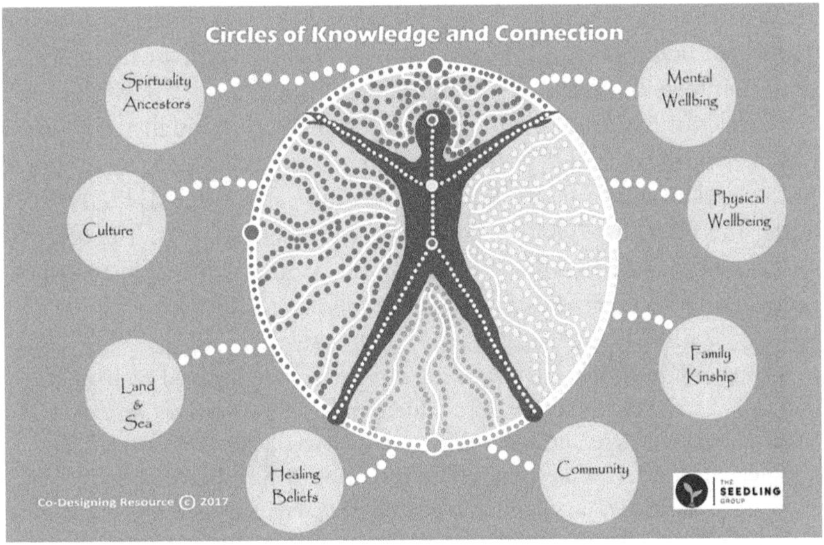


Fig. 7.2 Circles of Knowledge and Connection

***Kelleigh***: *I see saltwater men who are really active in their culture. They speak their languages, they dance, they've been through ceremony, but when they show up and we talk about anxiety, they say, "I've tried this mindfulness breathing stuff and it doesn't work". I suggest, "how about you try it at the beach, while you sit and listen to the waves? Remember you are your ancestors' dreams. Go and sit in that, feel the vibrations, stand in the water if you have to." They come back and say to me "that was incredible, how did you know that?" I say, "well, it's in your DNA." All those techniques like mindfulness are all about re-connecting. For me it speaks to how much we are displaced people on our own lands. We live in a world that privileges someone else's knowledge system; a system that disregards or is not interested in understanding what needs to be different to work for us.*

Remember to go back to Chap. 4 for Kelleigh's explanation of how she uses this model in her practice.

## The Five Rs of Trauma-Informed Care

The '5 Rs Model' (Fig. 7.3) is another holistic model that we use to guide trauma-informed practice in combination with the SEWB Wheel, and the Circles of Knowledge and Connection model. Originally this model was developed by the US government organisation SAMHSA (Substance Abuse and Mental Health Services Administration (SAMHSA, 2014) under the US Department of Health and Human Services. The original model had four Rs (Realise, Recognise, Respond and Resist re-traumatisation). SAMHSA defines the model as follows:

> A program, organization, or system that is trauma-informed **realizes** the widespread impact of trauma and understands potential paths for recovery; **recognizes** the signs and symptoms of trauma in clients, families, staff, and others involved with the system; and **responds** by fully integrating knowledge about trauma into policies, procedures, and practices, and seeks to actively **resist** re-traumatization (SAMHSA, 2014, p. 9).

Work that Aboriginal academic and traumatologist Judy Atkinson did with The Healing Foundation in different Aboriginal communities

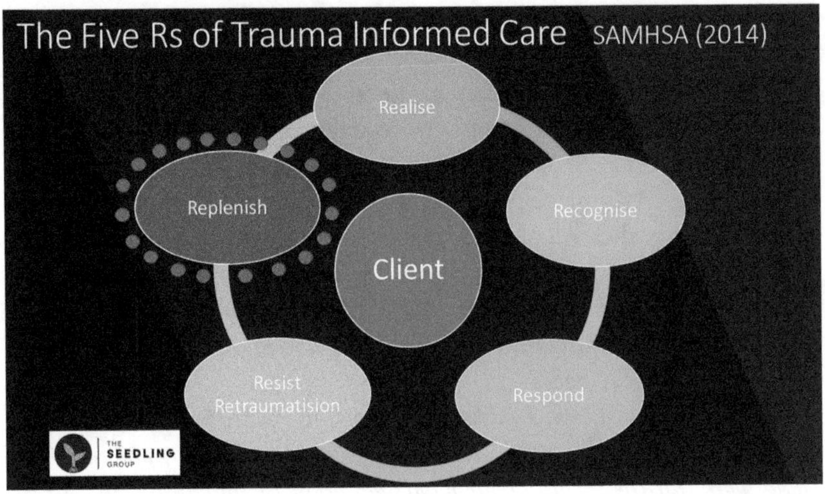


**Fig. 7.3** Five Rs of trauma informed care. Source: Adapted from SAMHSA (2014, p. 9)

influenced the addition of the 5th R, 'Replenish'. Replenishment refills or rebalances, an aspect that's missing from the original Four Rs model, which mainly focuses on recognising and responding. Replenishment helps us re-balance and care for each other, care for self and also care for Country. It is what's been in cultural practice since the beginning of our being. It's about being together, about supporting each other being on Country and grounding ourselves on earth and all we are connected to. Replenishment can bring about feelings of calm and true connection. It is about the songs and the dances, the ceremonies and protocols. Songs and dances replenish our cultural identity, while moving major muscle groups and changing neurochemicals, helping us burn through stress chemicals and rebalance our systems. That is what you need to do in trauma response work. See Chap. 8 for practical suggestions on using the 5th R to minimise vicarious trauma and compassion fatigue.

More recently a 6th R, *Regenerate and Revive* has been proposed (Cubillo, 2021), which we talk more about at the end of Chap. 9.

## The FEAR Rubric

Another useful model or 'rubric' we use in our practice, uses the acronym FEAR to identify four areas of behavioural adaptation following trauma (Evans & Coccoma, 2014). Based in neuroscience, the FEAR rubric enables us to recognise trauma responses. This can guide our choices in trauma-informed approaches. All of these challenging survival behaviours have been identified across cultures, which is why it's so effective and widely used.

***Nicole****: I like to think about this model as a way to make sure I'm working in a safe way with trauma clients. It makes it easy to remember the four elements of a trauma response.*

***Kelleigh****: In my work, I have found that this model brings together in a non-judgmental and accessible way all the parts of my therapy practice that I know work, all the theory about what's going on in your brain and all the neuroscience about neuroplasticity and synaptic pruning. The descriptions that follow are the way that I think about the domains of the FEAR rubric.*

## F is for Fear Extinction

Anyone who's experienced trauma may have trouble feeling safe again, may continue to feel their threat response, even when the threat is no longer there (Sehlmeyer et al., 2011). Think back to that image of the PTSD brain scan we look at in Chap. 4, showing cortisol scattered throughout the brain, compared with the scan of a healthy brain, where the cortisol was sitting where we expect to see it. The brain that has been affected by PTSD and flooded with cortisol is what keeps the traumatised person in a state of hyper-vigilance or hyper-arousal. There hasn't been a chance to expel the fear response and integrate new information. This leaves the whole system stuck, looking for threat.

## E is for Emotional Regulation

When you're stuck in your threat response, all those neuro chemicals that activate fight, flight, freeze or befriend are flooding in. This makes regulating your emotional response difficult, because you are misreading everything, looking for danger everywhere. It can look to others like overreaction. Someone might say something to you like "how are you today?" and you get angry and respond with "how the hell do you think I am?" Prolonged activation can result in exhaustion, a result of depletion of a balanced chemical response, leaving you depressed, fatigued, unresponsive and isolated.

## A is for Attentional Bias and Cognitive Distortion

If you have experienced early childhood trauma and found that the world is an unsafe place, then you will pay attention to information that confirms and reinforces that belief. Cognitively, you are only looking for things that confirm you are unsafe. Attentional bias can inadvertently place you in more danger because you don't read signs properly, or you overestimate the importance of signs or thoughts confirming your distorted belief. For example, if you have lost a loved one in hospital, you may avoid going to hospital because you believe it is an unsafe place because people die there.

Another source of these kinds of cognitive distortions to be alert to is when people have negative views of themselves. If someone grew up being told that there was something wrong with them," you're stupid" or "you're a bad kid", they integrate those negative messages into their knowledge system and worldview. Part of their knowledge system says that there's something wrong with them and that clearly, they're not as good as everyone else. When they make a mistake, that just confirms that there's something wrong with them. For example, they might get 80% on a test, and I tell them they did really well. Even though I'm saying they've done a great job, all they can hear is, "I got 20% of that wrong. What was my problem? Why didn't I perform?" They focus on the negative story, because it is the threat they've got built into their brain which just keeps reinforcing that story. It's very difficult to change those narratives, those stories. It's not just a matter of saying the new story over and over, like repeating affirmations, it's about building the new neural pathways or networks that need to be supported and maintained to avoid network pruning.

## R is for Relational Dysfunction

For all the reasons we've been talking about, when someone is still in a threat response from a previous trauma, it leaves them looking for threat, always reacting and never feeling safe, which can lead to anxiety, depression or other emotional challenges. This makes it difficult for them to form trusting relationships. This is very important to understand when you want to build trust with someone who's experienced trauma in your role as a practitioner or therapist. As practitioners, we have systems we work in where we might be assigned a particular number of sessions to work with this person. But a client who's experienced trauma is going to take a long time to trust you. They may have been in and out of the system before; they may have had interactions with it where it hasn't been very supportive or it's been retraumatising. This is particularly the case for First Nations Peoples who have the added trauma of everyday racism we talk about in Chap. 6. This is why some people can take a long time to seek help, because one of the things about having a brain that has experienced trauma is that you feel like you don't deserve help or that seeking help is risky for you and it's going to be a bad experience.

If you as a practitioner are still coming to understand trauma and its complexities, your client who has experienced trauma may take some time to trust and form a relationship with you. They will test you, they will be cautious before they feel they can trust you, "Will you be there? Will you stay there? Will you be able to cope with what I'm about to tell you? Will you follow through on the support that you said you're going to give me? If you say you're going to help me heal, will you actually stay the distance?" They know it is not a quick fix.

Another important thing to understand about working with relational dysfunction is that it's hard as a practitioner not to get caught up in moving to rescue your client. It's very uncomfortable to sit with someone who experiences trauma and not move to take away their power by 'fixing' them. It's back to understanding that if you try to fix someone, they're not being allowed to grow a new neural network themselves; they're not able to build their own skills and you're not helping them to build their capacity, which is what you want them to do to heal. One of the biggest challenges facing us as practitioners is *sitting with the discomfort*, therapeutically holding the client safe while they remember the experience and calm themselves.

## Culturally Safe, Trauma-Informed Practice Principles

These principles (Fig. 7.4) are holistic, acknowledging the importance of restorative and reciprocal approaches that guide us in our practice. They underpin the Five Rs of trauma-informed care. These principles are good to have on hand if you want to make sure you're working in a culturally safe and trauma-informed way, particularly with First Nations clients. We consider each of these principles in turn.

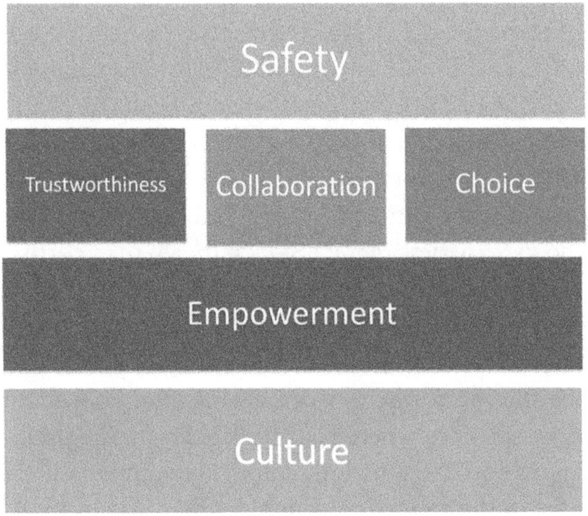


**Fig. 7.4** Trauma-informed practice principles. Source: Adapted from Harris & Fallot, (2001)

## Safety

Before reading this section, you might like to read Chap. 3, where we talk about why cultural safety is so important when you work in First Nations contexts.

A good way to begin in providing cultural safety for your clients is to think about the physical environment they will be walking in to. The actual physical environment itself gives our limbic system messages: *does it feel safe here?* Your client will be thinking, “Can I see that you understand or even know about my culture just from looking around this place? Can I see, hear and smell things that represent my culture?” Creating a space that is respectful and welcoming of your clients’ cultures is an important first step in ensuring they will feel safe. This could include: having local Indigenous art on the walls; burning bush medicine oils, especially flower essences (remember DNA recognises smells); and having food and drink available. These things give the message that First Nations cultures are privileged here.

A good team exercise is to get your team together and ask, “how can we make this place feel welcoming and safer for our clients?” Bring your collective attention to the question of what safety looks like here for you, your colleagues, your clients and for the community you work with. What do you need to change and extend on? For example, we know that bright fluorescent lights can be stimulating to the senses. If your client is someone who is experiencing PTSD, with all that cortisol sprinkled throughout the brain, the last thing you would want for them is to walk into an environment where the lights are glaring down on them and it’s sterile and uncomfortable.

It might be the room where you’re having your consultations. If that room has no windows or where your back is facing the door, your client may feel trapped in that situation. Another example is if the only sign your clients see in the room says something like, “aggression will not be tolerated”. A person who is hyper-aroused could be triggered when they see that and feel immediately attacked, which may feed into their cognitive distortion. Think about those things before your client comes in. Meeting them in that room may not be the safest thing for them.

There are other ways to address safety issues. It might mean thinking about your own physical safety. For example, if you're a nurse on night shift or doing outreach work, you'll want to know how you're going to be safe while you're working or walking to your car. It might relate to how you communicate, for example, if you are writing up reports, ask yourself questions like, "Am I keeping this information safe? Could this information be accessed by someone who shouldn't see it? Will this information be used against my client? Am I writing it in a safe way? Am I using 'othering' language? Am I using pathologising language or am I using strengths-based language?" These things all add up to a culture of working safely in your relationships with your clients.

## Trustworthiness

Trustworthiness is more than keeping your promises or letting people know in advance if you have to make a change to a meeting time. It's also things like not closing early, or if you say you're going to be open six days a week, don't just take the sixth day off without telling people. It's as simple as your client being confident that no one's ever going to know their information, that you have processes in place that are reliable and trustworthy. You can reassure them that you have systems that allow no one to share your information; you make agreements; you sign contracts; you let your client know often that you can be trusted with their information. If you can't promise that, you need to tell them that you may have to share their information so they can decide how and what they share with you.

***Kelleigh:*** *I always have to say to my clients, "you know, everything you say is confidential unless you indicate you are a threat to yourself or someone else".*

In small organisations where other family members might be working, confidentiality takes more consideration. Find out what your organisation's policies are in relation to cultural protocols relating to mandatory reporting and how they will keep their clients safe. If the client-therapist relationship can be maintained, mandatory reporting can be a safety measure, not a punitive act against your client.

Even more important for the client to know is that they can trust you not to react in an over-the-top way when they tell you about their trauma. They need to trust that you have the professional skills to know how to support and help them. That means making sure you're constantly upgrading your skills, that you are getting good supervision and support, as well as taking care of yourself so they can be reassured you have the resources and capabilities to support them. It also means not promising what you can't deliver. If you are out of your depth or feel you can't be of help, admit that. Recommend or bring in someone who has the skills and experience that can meet your client's needs. Trust is so hard to build and so quick to break. It's a very fragile thing, particularly for a person with a threat response system that's always on the lookout for danger. The moment there's any doubt about your ability to be trustworthy, that's the end of it.

## Collaboration

Cultural safety means working in partnerships. It's about not being the rescuer, it's not about being the expert of everything Aboriginal, someone who is going to 'fix' the community or the person you are going to work with. Collaboration means taking your knowledge and working with a client or community, with their unique knowledge and understanding, to see what solutions you can come up with together. That's completely different from going into a community, setting up shop and saying, "we're doing this, we can solve all your problems, come and see us". That very seldom works.

Collaboration is an absolute necessity if you're working with trauma clients. Trauma has multiple complexities, affecting many different parts of a person's life. For example, if you're working with a person who's experiencing homelessness and trauma, you will need to collaborate and form safe and trustworthy relationships with other relevant organisations. If you know you will be working with Indigenous clients, you must develop collaborative relationships with organisations you can safely refer to. This should be part of your practice from the beginning. Does this organisation welcome and understand Indigenous clients? How do you know that? If you don't know, you could contact your local Aboriginal medical centre or community Elders groups. It takes time and effort to form those relationships.

When you refer a client to someone you have a trustworthy relationship with this is what we call a 'soft handover'. A referral involves at a minimum, a conversation with the organisation you are referring to, in which you introduce the client you are referring. Without a soft handover, there's a risk that the safety link with the client can be broken. It's not uncommon for trauma clients to be referred on continually to different departments and organisations. Given how hard it is for someone who's experienced trauma to get themselves to the point of actually seeking help, it's very important that when you 'soft hand' them to another person, you are confident you can assure your client they're in safe hands. Tell the person "I know where you're going, I know this person, I'll be here when you come back", which is really saying, "I can speak for this person. I've checked out this organisation." It's a big responsibility. This is an essential component of trauma-informed care, even though it's not always easy to achieve in practice.

## Choice

We know that people with a trauma story have often had choice or control over the way they live their lives taken away from them. Offering a choice at every turn, no matter how seemingly small or insignificant, becomes a very important start to their healing. It might be as simple as, "Where would you like to meet? Would you like to meet in the office, or should we go for a walk on the beach, or should we meet under the tree, or in the park, or wherever else you would feel comfortable?" While this might work for the client, we often come up against system requirements like workplace health and safety. You might be required to say, "well, technically speaking, walking on the beach is not safe". This is another example of how working in a trauma-safe way may be inconsistent with some of the regulations of the workplace. But even within those constraints, we can still offer some simple choices, for example, offering a choice between a cup of tea or a coffee or a drink of water or a biscuit when they come into the room.

In the Scottish video about Trauma and the Brain we look at in Chap. 3, when the police say to the young woman "do you want a drink of water?", that helped to ground her. Even giving a choice as simple as what they would like to drink means the person has to problem solve, "I have to decide whether to have a drink or I have to work out which cup or what I want in my cup", all those simple acts move the person out of their emotional brain into their thinking, problem-solving brain.

If you're reading this and thinking, "that sounds easy, but that's not how our organisation works or that's not how practice works", there are still ways you can work within the constraints of workplace rules and regulations with a trauma-informed lens. For example, you might have arranged to have six sessions every Friday morning with your client. Then your client rings you one Friday morning and says, "I've been up with my family all night and I can't get out of bed and, quite frankly, I don't care about your appointment". If I were to respond in a trauma-informed way, I'd say, "okay, I understand that. Let's just reschedule this appointment". This might not be the policy of the workplace, but I can still decide to make a priority of giving my client the safety of making a choice based on what's good for them and what works for them.

Without choice, they may not show up, or if they do, they are less likely to feel okay about being there. They may not have the capacity to interact with you and it is likely you won't do anything that actually helps them. They'll just be meeting *your* needs, and what you're actually doing is igniting that threat response all over again. Any work you had done in an effort to calm that threat response will be lost. Asking them to commit when they feel threatened to do so is ultimately counterproductive.

## Empowerment

Empowerment means identifying your client's strengths as a person and inviting them to work with those strengths rather than trying to rescue them. Empowerment can mean being guided by your client, for example, offering them information and resources at a pace that suits them. Empowerment allows the client to integrate what they're learning into their knowledge system and to grow as a person as they build on their capacities, their identity, and their self-worth.

## Culture

The principle of 'culture' in trauma-informed practice encompasses all aspects of a person's identity: race; ethnicity; gender identity; sexual orientation; age; religion; spirituality; and connection to Country. If you're working with Indigenous people, the principle of 'culture' means seeking out every opportunity to incorporate culture into the way you work with your client or community. It could mean finding out everything about the community your client comes from, or the community you're about to work in; everything about the language, the historical journey, and trauma story of that community before you start work. For example, having the map of all the different language groups of Indigenous Peoples in Australia up on your wall (see Chap. 2) tells your client "you know something about my culture".

***Nicole:*** *I was yarning with a non-Indigenous colleague who was doing outreach work. He asked me, "when I'm working with people who are on the street and experiencing homelessness, is it okay for me to wear a pin of an Aboriginal and Torres Strait flag or does that just feel a bit fake?" My response is "if you're wearing a pin, it is likely that that person will look at you and say, "they know something about my culture, maybe this person is going to be safe".*

# Concluding Comments

While we hear policymakers say, "we need everything to be trauma-informed", there'll be a major public announcement about a policy that's definitely *not* trauma-informed. For example, following the findings of the Royal Commission into Institutional Responses to Child Sexual Abuse, the Australian Government announced that victims who had a criminal record would be ineligible to apply for compensation under the National Redress Scheme, even though there were strong links between offending and the trauma of their early abuse.[2] While there appears that

[2] See https://www.abc.net.au/news/2017-12-16/royal-commission-government-criticised-for--blocking-jail-redress/9264970#:~:text=Under the proposed national redress scheme, child sexual, fraud offences would also be barred from applying.

some awareness that trauma-informed practice is important, we're still not seeing it woven into our policies and our procedures. This is problematic because national and state laws, systems and structures continue to traumatise Aboriginal and Torres Strait Islander Peoples.

Aboriginal and Torres Strait Islander practitioners work within systems and frameworks that don't give us time to build those trusting and empowering relationships. We might be feeding information into a database or reporting system where there's no code for building relationships or spending time in community. How do you record all of that work you're doing and have that work validated? How do you then apply for funding, or have your program re-funded, if you're not acknowledged for that important part of your work? We've got systems that don't fit our social and emotional wellbeing framework or support trauma-informed practice. Australian systems that were supposedly set up for us as Aboriginal and Torres Strait Islander Peoples, often work against us, because they reflect non-Indigenous values and ways of operating. We've got to start thinking about how to change this system, in a way that at least allows us to record the work we do that contributes to genuine healing for First Nations trauma survivors.

For more information on trauma-informed care and practices, check out some of the extra readings at the end of this chapter.

**Activity 6.3 Check-out and Reflection**

Take a moment, check in with your body, feel what's happening in your body, think of a word that describes how you're feeling.

Take some time to write answers to these reflective questions:

- What do you think are the main differences between the biomedical health model and the SEWB wheel?
- In what ways do these different perspectives change the way you think about your own sense of wellbeing?
- Reflect on your own story of trauma in your life or in the life of your family. In what ways does the FEAR rubric help you make sense of that story?
- What would you need to change in your practice or at your workplace to make it more culturally safe?

## References and Further Reading


Cubillo, C. (2021). Trauma-informed care: Culturally responsive practice working with Aboriginal and Torres Strait Islander communities. *InPsych, 43*(3). Retrieved from https://psychology.org.au/for-members/publications/inpsych/2021/august-special-issue-3/trauma-informed-care

Donaldson, W. (2018). *Trauma-informed care: Literature scan.* Te Pou o te Whakaaro Nui.

Dudgeon, P., Milroy, H., & Walker, R. (2014). *Working together: Aboriginal and Torres Strait Islander mental health and wellbeing principles and practice* (2nd ed.). Commonwealth of Australia.

Dudgeon, P., & Holland, C. (2018). Recent developments in suicide prevention among the Indigenous peoples of Australia. *Australasian Psychiatry, 26*(2), 166–169. https://doi.org/10.1177/1039856218757637

Elliott, A., McIlwaine, F., Stone, N., & Proctor, K. (2015). *Aboriginal family therapy training program: Impact analysis report.* The Lowitja Institute.

Elliott, D. E., Bjelajac, P., Fallot, R. D., Markoff, L. S., & Reed, B. G. (2005). Trauma-informed or trauma-denied: Principles and implementation of trauma-informed services for women. *Journal of Community Psychology, 33*(4), 461–477. https://doi.org/10.1002/jcop.20063

Evans, A., & Coccoma, P. (2014). *Trauma-informed care: How neuroscience influences practice.* Routledge.

Gee, G., Dudgeon, P., Schultz, C., Hart, A., & Kelly, K. (2014). Aboriginal and Torres Strait Islander social and emotional wellbeing. In P. Dudgeon, H. Milroy, & R. Walker (Eds.), *Working together: Aboriginal and Torres Strait Islander mental health and wellbeing principles and practice* (pp. 55–68). Commonwealth of Australia.

Green, G. (2011). Developing trauma training for an Indigenous community: Hopefully not seagulls. *Australian Social Work, 64*(2), 215–227. https://doi.org/10.1080/0312407x.2010.518243

Hanson, R. F., & Lang, J. (2016). A critical look at trauma-informed care among agencies and systems serving maltreated youth and their families. *Child Maltreatment, 21*(2), 95–100. https://doi.org/10.1177/1077559516635274

Harris, M., & Fallot, R. D. (Eds.). (2001). *Using trauma theory to design service systems.* Jossey-Bass/Wiley.

Jennings, A. (2004). *Models for developing trauma-informed behavioral health systems and trauma-specific services.* National Association of State Mental Health Program Directors & National Technical Assistance Center for State Mental Health Planning.

Johnson, S. (2014). Knucwénte-kuc re Stsmémelt.s-kuc: Trauma-informed education for Indigenous children in foster care. *Canadian Social Work Review, 31*(2), 155–174.

Kelly, K., Dudgeon, P., Gee, G., & Glaskin, B. (2009). *Living on the Edge: Social and emotional wellbeing and risk and protective factors for serious psychological distress among Aboriginal and Torres Strait Islander people.* Cooperative Research Centre for Aboriginal Health.

Kezelman, C., & Stavropoulos, P. (2012). *Practice guidelines for treatment of complex trauma and trauma informed care and service delivery.* Blue Knot Foundation.

Kezelman, C. A., & Stavropoulos, P. (2016). *Trauma and the law: Applying trauma-informed practice to legal and judicial contexts.* Blue Knot Foundation.

Leitch, L. (2017). Action steps using ACEs and trauma-informed care: A resilience model. *Health & Justice, 5*(5), 1–10. https://doi.org/10.1186/s40352-017-0050-5

Muskett, C. (2014). Trauma-informed care in inpatient mental health settings: A review of the literature. *International Journal of Mental Health Nursing, 23*(1), 51–59. https://doi.org/10.1111/inm.12012

Quadara, A., & Hunter, C. (2016). *Principles of trauma-informed approaches to child sexual abuse: A discussion paper (1925289869).* Royal Commission into Institutional Responses to Child Sexual Abuse.

Randall, M., & Haskell, L. (2013). Trauma-informed approaches to law: Why restorative justice must understand trauma and psychological coping. *Dalhousie Law Journal, 36*(2), 501–534.

Raphael, B., & Swan, P. (1995). *"Ways Forward": National Consultancy Report on Aboriginal and Torres Strait Islander Mental Health.* Australian Government Publishing Service.

Sehlmeyer, C., Dannlowski, U., Schöning, S., Kugel, H., Pyka, M., Pfleiderer, B., Zwitserlood, P., Schiffbauer, H., Heindel, W., & Arolt, V. (2011). Neural correlates of trait anxiety in fear extinction. *Psychological Medicine, 41*(4), 789–798.

Substance Abuse and Mental Health Services Administration (SAMHSA). (2014). *SAMHSA's concept of trauma and guidance for a trauma-informed approach.* Retrieved from https://ncsacw.samhsa.gov/userfiles/files/SAMHSA_Trauma.pdf

The Lowitja Institute. (2019). *The First Response project: Trauma and culturally informed approaches to primary health care for women who experience violence.* Melbourne.

Wilson, A., Hutchinson, M., & Hurley, J. (2017). Literature review of trauma-informed care: Implications for mental health nurses working in acute inpatient settings in Australia. *International Journal of Mental Health Nursing, 26*(4), 326–343. https://doi.org/10.1111/inm.12344

# 8

# The Cost of Caring: Vicarious Trauma and Compassion Fatigue

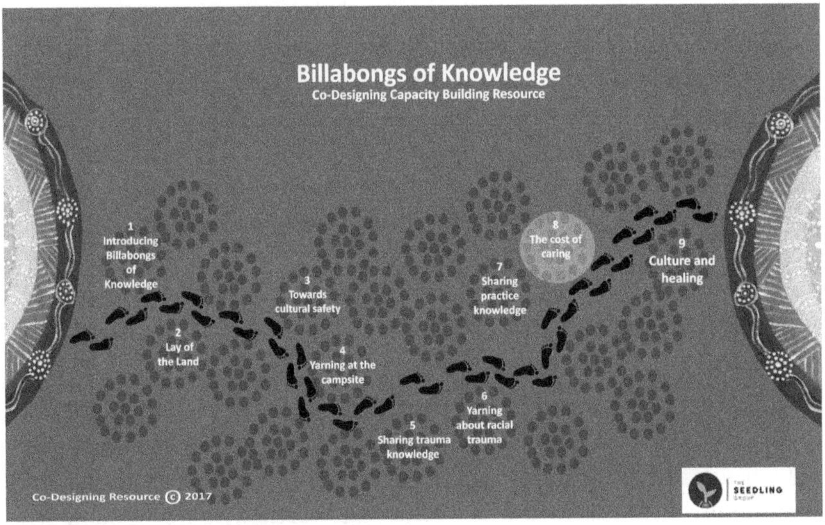


We acknowledge the traditional owners, the custodians of the land that we're meeting on today. We pay our respects to Elders, past, present and emerging and thank them for the wonderful custodianship of their lands. We ask you take a moment to reflect on whose Country you are on wherever you are reading this book.



N. Tujague, K. Ryan, *Cultural Safety in Trauma-Informed Practice from a First Nations Perspective*, https://doi.org/10.1007/978-3-031-13138-7_8

*During the Royal Commission into Institutional Responses to Child Sexual Abuse established in 2013, Aboriginal and Torres Strait Islander people were called upon to tell their stories. These experiences were difficult to talk about and many had never told their stories before because of the hurt and pain still impacting their lives and the lives of their families. This is the story of one incredibly strong Aboriginal woman, a survivor of the Stolen Generations, whose lived experience and cultural integrity made her a safe and trusted person to hear those stories. Although she was part of a team, people would wait and ask to talk to her. Despite official debriefing and professional supervision, after some years, she knew she was burning out, but she also carried the privilege and the burden of cultural responsibility. Many of those hearing the stories, including legal staff, burned out and suffered vicarious trauma. This woman's cultural load, her cultural responsibility was always present for her. She knew that if survivors didn't have someone they felt safe with to tell their stories to, they wouldn't have their truth told; they couldn't hold the perpetrators to account; they couldn't be part of the redress scheme set up to compensate survivors. Having a lived experience made this woman a safe and trusted person to hear these stories, however there was a huge personal cost for her caring.*

## Introduction

At this billabong we yarn about what happens when you are exposed to the trauma experienced by others and how you can minimise the potential harms of that exposure. Various terms have been used to describe the symptoms that affect front-line workers and carers who treat people who have suffered trauma. These include 'compassion fatigue', 'vicarious trauma, 'vicarious PTSD' and 'burnout'. Remember it's a normal threat response; it's not *if* it will happen, but *when*. While a single, overarching term for these symptoms has not been agreed upon, the way you respond is the same: after every battle you must wash off the blood and attend to your wounds before you start again. To do this, you need to be aware that when you are listening to someone's trauma story, you are carrying that extra weight of holding the space for them. Depending on the type of exposure and the resources you have available to you, the impact will look different. This is what this chapter is about: *the cost of being in the battle of truth-telling* and what you can do to minimise the impact of vicarious

**Activity 8.1 Check-in**

Again, this is an opportunity to bring your mind and body together to bring yourself into the present. So just take a moment to feel what's happening in your body. What is your body telling your brain? Think of a feeling word, like 'glad', 'sad', 'anxious' or 'excited'. Notice if your words tend to be thinking words like 'interested', 'grateful' or 'annoyed', rather than feeling words. Connect in, bring yourself to the here and now. That will take your brain to a place where hopefully you can take on lots of good information without getting too overloaded. Breathe deeply and ask yourself, "how do I feel when I am exposed to stories of trauma?"

trauma and compassion fatigue. We finish the chapter looking at the ethical imperative of self-care strategies, encompassed within the 5th R of trauma-informed practice: 'Replenish'.

## Responding to Trauma Stories: Empathy or Sympathy?

We hear frontline service providers and mental health staff talk about 'armouring up' (McGrath & Reavey, 2016). Armouring up is necessary to prepare yourself to be empathetic. Armouring up is consciously preparing, with the tools and skills you have, to hear trauma stories and be present. Remember to de-armour before returning to your family and friends by checking out and debriefing. You can be empathetic without being armoured up, but you are at more risk of being injured. Having empathy means being able to put yourself in the place of that person, *feeling through* their experience with them and holding them and you safe.

It's important to understand the difference between empathy and sympathy, because one is much more effective in helping someone through trauma than the other. We think of empathy as 'feeling with' someone, while sympathy is feeling 'sorry for' a person. Watch this clever animation by Brené Brown[1] who explains that while empathy *fuels connection*, sympathy *drives disconnection* (Fig. 8.1).

[1] https://www.youtube.com/watch?v=1Evwgu369Jw

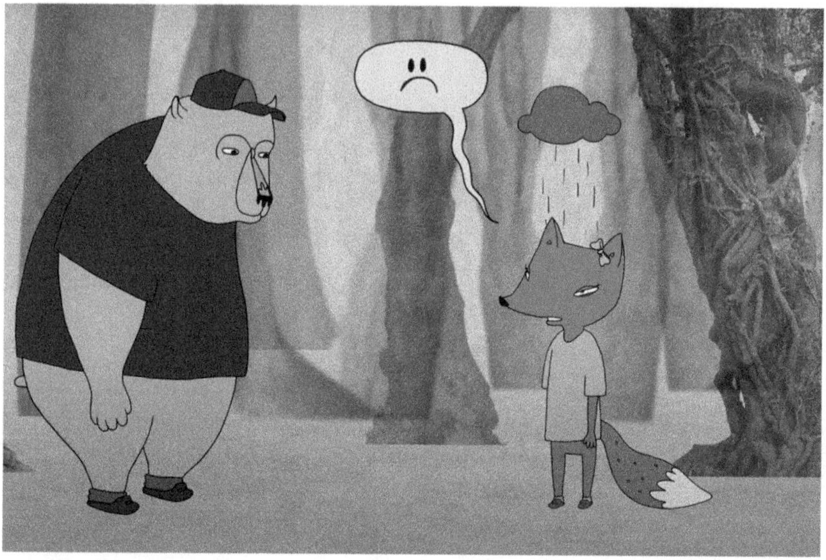

Fig. 8.1 Brené Brown video on empathy

**Activity 8.2 Reflections on the Brené Brown Video**

Source: RSA Shorts: Brené Brown on Empathy Illustrator: Katy Davis (aka Gobblynne).

- What was the most important thing you got out of the video?
- Do you act out of sympathy or empathy and can you tell the difference?
- Are you more likely to be the antelope or the bear?

***Kelleigh**: The main thing I got out of this clip was I couldn't think of a better way to explain what's happening when someone is being empathetic.*

***Nicole**: I really love it when she says, "You don't have to make it better." I think because I'm a natural rescuer, I always want to make it better. I can't even remember how many people I've given that line to, "I'm just so glad you told me", and how many times I've used it myself. It's really powerful as it takes you straight out of rescuing or sympathy into, "okay, I'm just sitting in this hole with you and I'm glad you told me."*

When you work empathetically with someone who has experienced trauma, you move into the space where you are at risk of vicarious trauma.

## Vicarious Trauma: Not If, But When

For a lot of people who work with trauma, the statement that 'vicarious trauma is a certainty' can be very confronting. Our understanding of neuroscience confirms that it really *is* 'not if, but when'. We have come to see that we can minimise the risks of developing vicarious trauma, sometimes thought of as 'contagious trauma' (Coddington, 2017), which we go into a bit later in the chapter. The neurobiology of trauma tells us that when you hear someone's trauma story, or you're working with trauma stories, or you see something traumatic on television, or even when you're *reading* a trauma story, you will have a threat response.

***Nicole:*** *When I watch a scary movie and I'm really involved in the plot, even though my brain knows 'this is just a movie', my body still goes into a threat response. I can get really scared, my heart starts to pound, my mouth goes dry. That's my body going into a type of vicarious trauma response. They reckon the worst thing you can watch is torture. It has its own special movie rating. It can be the same when you watch the news, which is even worse, because it's real.*

Think of vicarious trauma as repetitive small doses or small activations of threat response. If your job is to listen to or read about, or work in other ways with, the trauma story, such as administrators, journalists or lawyers (Hassing & Quayle, 2019), then you'll also be getting repetitive activations.

When you work with a client who's sharing their trauma story and you're helping them make sense of it, they get to cry, they get to be angry, and you help them regulate; you help them work through that story. They get to release that emotion and chemical, make sense of the story, recover and move on. But when they leave, you're often still flooded with that neuro-chemical your body has produced in response to hearing or reading the trauma story. We as workers get paid to hold ourselves together while we listen to those stories. *That is the deal.*

While we might show some emotion, we don't collapse into a mess. We hold you to that point where you can heal, to that level of activation where it can get challenging, and we support you to be present and hold the space safe so you can process it and move on. Then when the client leaves, we might think, 'okay, that was hard!' We are left with the residue chemical in our bodies, whereas the client no longer has it in theirs, because they got to cry and shake it out. We are looking for fear extinction, to move into a memory, not a response. To do that you have to be exposed to the stimulus, feel the emotion, be held in safety so you can give context to it and then it is no longer stuck, waiting to activate.

It's one thing to hear a whole lot of facts and try to remember them like you would in a classroom situation, but it's quite another when you listen to a story. Indigenous Peoples have used this explanation of why storywork (Archibald, 2008) is so powerful. Your brain does this amazing thing where it creates all these images and all this context as you listen. You imagine people doing things in the story, you can visualise the place where it's happening. It's taking on that full context that lays down those deep neural networks that are designed to help us to remember things. This is also why vicarious trauma happens (McCann & Pearlman, 1990).

## Vicarious PTSD

***Kelleigh***: *I used to supervise a therapist who worked with children who had been physically and sexually abused. After some time, they realised they were starting to have dreams that had the exact same imagery in them. Memories of those stories would just come to them in an intrusive and unexpected way. This is when the experience becomes vicarious PTSD, or secondary or acquired trauma (Adams et al.,* 2006; *Rauvola et al.,* 2019; *Reuben,* 2015*). The therapist chose to protect their wellbeing by stopping that work.*

Deep hurt, whether individual or collective, has emotion and energy. If you are a First Nations person who is working with people who have the same collective or lived experience, while your worldview makes you the best person for the job because you understand and are more likely to be a safe person for your client, it also makes you quite vulnerable to the risks and harms associated with vicarious PTSD. So many First Nations Peoples who work in this space choose to leave their jobs because the system fails to protect them against vicarious trauma and/or vicarious PTSD, or makes *them* responsible for minimising the harm. When vicarious trauma is a workplace risk, it is the *employer's* responsibility to protect their staff.

An example is when an Indigenous worker listens to a story about sexual abuse that happened in an institution and then they realise their grandmother was at that institution. All of a sudden, they understand their grandmother's behaviour and its intergenerational impact. So, what does the worker do with that anger and grief? When they understand that this experience is part of a natural response to an unnatural event, they can seek professional help. Be aware that when vicarious PTSD overlaps with different traumas, in this case intergenerational trauma, it is often difficult to diagnose and detect. When you identify compounding traumas, you understand the need to work in a holistic way.

## Compassion Fatigue

'Compassion fatigue' as defined by Charles Figley (1995), considered the first person to use that term, encompasses both vicarious trauma and burnout. Figley studied what was happening with support staff and frontline workers while they were treating trauma victims, especially in disasters. The whole reasoning behind his research was to argue that compassion fatigue and vicarious trauma should be treated like any other workplace risk. When this research initially came out, Figley's evidence of compassion fatigue was used against individual workers. Their employers would say things like, "you're no longer fit for your job, you need to be moved on," or, "you can't do your job". It was seen as an individual deficit and used as a weapon against workers.

## Burnout

While vicarious trauma and compassion fatigue have similar aspects, burnout is different, as it can happen even when you are not dealing with traumatised clients. Burnout can occur when you have a workload that you can never get on top of, have too many meetings to attend, too many reports to write, or all of those things about your job that you perceive are not beneficial to your clients; they are not actually helping you achieve your clients' goals. It's all those other things that pull you away, that you can never get done, because they're continually adding up, to the point where you reach a level of exhaustion, that is similar to a trauma response (Roche et al., 2013; Parker et al., 2021; Leiter, 2018).

There is often an overlap between vicarious trauma and burnout. In Australia and in many countries, mental health or helping services are underfunded and therefore understaffed. It's not uncommon for workers to have a higher workload than they can attend to. While you might assume that someone working in a trauma context has compassion fatigue or vicarious trauma, it may well be burnout, or a combination of both.

The important thing here is that the pathways to recovery for burnout and vicarious trauma are different—similar, but different, and if you only attend to one, you will miss key elements of the other.

## Warning Signs of and Risk Factors for Compassion Fatigue and Vicarious Trauma

The first signs of compassion fatigue and vicarious trauma can be *disconnection*, from self and from support networks. For First Nations Peoples, the disconnection can also be from cultural practice and from spiritual connections, including listening to ancestral voices. This is why we emphasise connecting mind, body and spirit as part of checking-in.

Sometimes the early signs of compassion fatigue and vicarious trauma are first recognised in the body. They can manifest as headaches, backache, migraines, fatigue, and stomach and digestive problems. Early signs can also appear in your thoughts, such as distorted thinking, negative automatic thoughts or paranoia. You might have thoughts like, "this work doesn't affect me", "why can't I help my client?", "I can't solve this", "I can't switch off" or "I'm so tired all the time". When your system becomes overwhelmed, you move into hyper-arousal. It's that not being able to switch off; it's that adrenaline and cortisol pumping through your body and you're not attending to it. You go into that space where you have the brake on and the accelerator on at the same time, which leads to exhaustion or hypo-arousal. This can put you at risk of developing anxiety, depression and cognitive distortion (Foa & Kozak, 1986).

Feelings you might experience include worthlessness, hopelessness, not being good enough, lack of self-efficacy (Bandura, 1997), general anxiety or even anger or rage. Some of the behaviours might include crying a lot (or not being able to cry), overeating, avoidance or procrastination, sleeping a lot without feeling refreshed or coping strategies such as problematic use of alcohol or other drugs. Common behaviours might include fighting, arguing, overreacting and cynicism, for example, "what's the point, they are only going to do it again, it doesn't matter how much I try".

Risk factors that influence compassion fatigue and vicarious trauma are many and varied. They include *organisational* risk factors. Our mainstream systems continue to reward the worker who delivers beyond what should be expected of them or is reasonable for their wellbeing. Occupational stressors include those obligations that you cannot possibly meet without either working in your own time or not looking after yourself. Support for workers' wellbeing needs to be written into your workplace policies, rules and regulations. While most organisations put in place policies and procedures to cover situations that arise in the workplace, without having a trauma-informed understanding and human resources staff who have been trained in cultural safety, those policies and processes become ineffective at best or weaponised at worst, blunt instruments that continue to do harm.

Compassion fatigue can also be felt at an organisational level. Unfortunately, what can happen with organisations that are fatigued is they start to become punitive, which puts more pressure on their staff.

***Nicole:*** *I worked for an organisation that was very taxing on its employees. They would put in long hours, travel for long stretches of time at the expense of their personal lives and were often expected to use their own homes and cars as part of their role. These people gave so much for their jobs because they were invested in the wellbeing of their trauma clients. Then when someone bought a coffee on the company card on their way home from an extended work trip to a remote area, it triggered a severe reprimand from head office, putting* *their job in jeopardy. This inflexibility and lack of give and take was distressing for the employees who were being punished for the organisation's fatigue.*

Especially under pressure are First Nations organisations that are often established to service priority populations[2], such as people who've come into contact with the criminal justice system or are experiencing unemployment or continuous housing hardship. These service providers are often under-funded and therefore under-staffed. Pressures like these can put organisations at risk of compassion fatigue.

Using 'lived experience' voices has become crucial in building meaningful policy and programs however, the risk for a lived experience participant is triggering any ongoing or unresolved trauma. The responsibility lies with the service provider to support and care for these participants. You may be living with an unresolved trauma and working with a client who has a similar trauma story. Continuing to work with that client without listening to the warning signs of your body, makes you vulnerable to retraumatisation and at risk of vicarious trauma. You may also experience vicarious trauma if you are a researcher listening to trauma stories (Eades et al., 2020).

***Kelleigh**: I worked with some Indigenous researchers who didn't know why they were coming undone after listening to their participants' trauma stories. They didn't know why their spirit felt heavy, why they were getting unwell and stressed and cranky. It was because the stories of trauma they were listening to for their research were also <u>their</u> own collective trauma stories. They were being triggered, and their bodies were remembering.*

The problem with having unresolved trauma is not only that it makes you more vulnerable. As a practitioner, if I have unresolved trauma that I either don't know about or haven't worked on, that will affect my capacity to attend to my client and keep them safe. Normally when I'm working with you as a client in therapy and I hear that change in your voice when you mention something, or I notice your reaction to something, these are the signs that tell me I need to explore the unconscious reaction that lies behind that physical action. But if I have unresolved trauma that is similar or close to your trauma story, I'm not going there, not only because I don't even *know* to go there but because my alarm system is also going off. We often say, "*you can't take someone where you've never been*".

[2] With the move away from deficit language, the term 'priority populations' is preferred over the term 'vulnerable populations' (Munari et al., 2021).

## What Helps Minimise Vicarious Trauma and Compassion Fatigue?

***Kelleigh:*** *One of our colleagues who is a First Nations Elder, works for an organisation that supports Aboriginal and Torres Strait Islander clients who have experienced trauma. The organisation has made Fridays a day where she has no commitments. She can take the day to replenish; she can use the time in whatever way will support her social and emotional wellbeing. She says this means she is likely to stay with the workplace because it reduces her vicarious trauma, making this trauma work sustainable.*

### Compassion Satisfaction

***Kelleigh:*** *An organisation may have a receptionist who is trauma-informed and the first point of contact for people visiting the organisation, people who may be traumatised and acting out. The receptionist completes the intake, hears part of the story, sees the person in their pain, is compassionate and gentle with them, while taking all of their necessary details. They then hand them on to the doctor or the therapist. A culturally safe and trauma-informed organisation might incorporate appropriate ways for the receptionist and relevant staff to be kept informed about the progress of clients they have met at the front desk.*

Compassion satisfaction is one way to reduce compassion fatigue (Sodeke-Gregson et al., 2013). The 'cloak of silence' that ensures our clients' confidentiality often means there is no feedback loop in the system that lets all staff understand how their input has made a difference. At the neurological level, when you hear someone's story of trauma, you become activated; when you can follow that story and understand that your contribution helped that person, you receive a neurochemical reward that comes with compassion satisfaction. It also gives you personal benefits, such as self-efficacy, a belief you can change things for the better, and therefore feel safer in your environment. You get positive reinforcement that you've done something good.

## Workplace Support

While compassion satisfaction is very influential in minimising the impact of compassion fatigue, so is workplace support. This is knowing that you work with people who believe in the same course you are taking or are working towards the same goals as you are. It's the support you get from your colleagues and from your workplace (Sprang et al., 2007; Stamm, 2002). This is particularly apparent in a workplace that is trauma-informed, where that workplace support is embedded in policies and processes as well as in the working environment. It is about making sure that people receive appropriate supervision and get the training they need to do their job. It is about ensuring your colleagues are supported and that the organisation supports you as a whole group. This means involvement in group debriefings; group outings and events that build cohesion; and acknowledgement from the organisation that work-life balance is critical for staff to do the best job possible for their clients.

## Connection

Connection most commonly means connection to meaningful relationships, but it can also refer to other social and emotional wellbeing areas on the Social and Emotional Wellbeing Wheel, like connection to Country, connection to spirit, connection to family and kinship, connection to culture. This is why making sure you have culturally appropriate group supervision and feeling like you belong in a healthy, culturally safe workplace, is critically important in minimising vicarious trauma and compassion fatigue.

If you're in a work situation where you're not getting that support, for example, where all the language is deficit language, the workplace culture is fatigued, no one is connecting, where everyone is operating in silos and just surviving, you could explore these steps:

- increase your awareness of protective factors
- find a support network
- suggest changes based on the current knowledge we have about the signs that indicate the dangers of vicarious trauma

- use the empirical knowledge we have about what lies behind compassion fatigue and vicarious trauma
- take this information to the people who can change the systems and say, "we need to look after ourselves in a better way so that the work we do is sustainable".

If you can't influence the decision makers, the best you can do is minimise the impact of the stress of working there. If you are aware that you are in a highly activated state, go home and do something that replenishes you and uses up that stress chemical. Remember when there's no escape, there's only minimisation. Compassion is only complete when it includes compassion for yourself.

## The 5th R: Replenish

To end this chapter, we unpack that fifth R of trauma-informed care, 'Replenish', which we mentioned at the last billabong. Replenishing is all about self-care, one of the most important things you can do to minimise the inevitable impacts of vicarious trauma and compassion fatigue. For many First Nations Peoples replenishment was always part of rebalancing the collective after a journey or after a major event.

### Self-Care as Ethical Imperative

What is so important to understand is that self-care is actually an *ethical imperative*. There's a book you can have a look at called *Fit to Practice* (Frankcom et al., 2016), which says if you're not self-caring, if you're not operating to the best of your ability, then you're not doing the best you can for your client. You would need to ask yourself, ethically, "should I be doing this? Is it okay to give my client sub-optimal support, not the best I can give?" If you're working with trauma clients and practising methods like 'Brainspotting' (Grand, 2013) or EMDR, which stands for 'Eye Movement Desensitization and Reprocessing' (Shapiro & Brown, 2019), treatments that work with complex trauma, then you'll know that if you're not functioning at your best, you'll probably be missing things you could be attending to in your work with your client (Pearlman & Caringi, 2009).

***Nicole:*** *I love this idea of self-care as ethical imperative. When I give a lecture at university, if I haven't slept properly, or if I haven't given myself some time to think through my concepts and the stories I want to use, I'm not really giving my students everything. I haven't really self-cared, and when I self-care, that's what makes me work in such a better way.*

***Kelleigh:*** *You're probably reading this and thinking "but who has a perfect life?" Most days, I do just drag myself in there after I've dealt with home and the kids. If I'm coming to work exhausted because life happened when I went home last night, I know I'm not going to be my best today. If I own that and say, "okay, I'm going to support myself today to be the best I can be with where I am and the resources I have", I am in charge of my own self-care. To be clear, I'm not saying if you're not giving your best then you shouldn't be doing your job, I'm saying it's important to <u>know</u> that if you're not taking care of yourself, you will probably not be working at your best. It's about being honest with yourself and putting some resources in place that can support you, instead of beating yourself up and pushing yourself harder. You're not doing the wrong thing if you prioritise your self-care.*

***Nicole:*** *I've got a bit of a problem with self-care though, Kell. I understand why it's really important and I understand the neuroscience behind it, but I feel like we work in a system that rewards us <u>not</u> to practice self-care. Can you imagine saying to your boss on a busy Friday afternoon, "I'm leaving early because I'm going to have a massage"? I mean, who does that? Because if you work harder, stay behind, do the extra bit, and you're a type A personality who's competitive and goes after the promotion, our systems will reward you. This makes self-care even harder.*

## Everyday Self-Care Minimises Everyday Exposure to Trauma

Practising self-care creates an environment of safety which is the first step towards minimising vicarious trauma and compassion fatigue. There's a whole industry described as 'self-care', as we know, but to practice *real* self-care, it's not simply the big bubble bath, the big holiday, the one-off retreat. While they are all great things, effective self-care involves *everyday actions*. It means constantly refilling that cup of joy. A lot of the things you do may have started out as *feeling like* self-care, for example, little rewards like having that extra glass of wine. Your self-care may have crept into things that are really *distractions*, like binge-watching a television series or constantly checking social media. Everyday self-care actions are made up of rituals and habits that continually allow you to be well and help minimise vicarious trauma: eating the right foods for your body; moving your body; connecting to people and the environment which are good for your spirit.

## Listening to Your Body

When you stop listening to your body, your body and your stress will show up in other ways. We often ask: "what's your body telling you?" When we check in with you, we say: "where do you feel it? Give it a name … what's the feeling?" We know that if you are experiencing trauma or high levels of stress, it's not uncommon to have stomach aches or headaches or neck pain. Remember there's a whole field of research that looks at where emotions show up in the body, as we talk about in Chap. 2.

For example, you might think that you're doing okay, but when you think about it a bit more, you realise: "actually, I've had indigestion for the last six months. It's just because I drink too much coffee." You need to ask yourself: "*why* am I drinking too much coffee?" You need to peel back where that came from:

You might start by asking yourself:

*Q: "What's the story of you drinking too much coffee? When did you start drinking too much coffee?"*

*A: "When I became too tired to do my work".*

*Q: "So you're drinking too much coffee because you are tired. Why are you tired?"*

*A: "I'm not sleeping well."*

*Q: "Why aren't you sleeping well?"*

*A: "I'm worried about my workload and the horrible things that have happened to the people I see. I don't get good sleep and I wake up tired, the caffeine in the coffee helps me cope with being tired."*

So where does this story really start? Does it start with the coffee or does it start with the vicarious trauma? While the coffee may be a contributing factor, remember that too much stress hormone stops you digesting your food. It decides, "oh, we've got to run from the crocodile, we don't need to digest lunch." It's about understanding the source of your discomfort, through listening to what your body is telling you.

## Making Time for Your Support Systems

Drawing on support outside your work is critical if you are constantly exposed to trauma. In Chap. 4 we talked about how your sense of what's healthy in terms of your own wellbeing changes when you are constantly in threat response. For example, the paramedic who says 'nothing shocks me anymore'. If you're stressed or working with complex trauma all day, you start to think that feeling of hyperarousal is your 'normal'. You don't have any way to rebalance or recheck where you are in the Window of Tolerance. Think of the police officer who's out there dealing with crimes and all sorts of crises every day. If they are constantly dealing with young people who are being harmed and go home to their own children, they may not let their kids leave their sight, because now it feels to them that the world is not safe for children. That's what we call a type of *cognitive distortion,* a major warning sign of vicarious trauma. It's showing that your point of reference has changed from a more normal, balanced viewpoint to measuring everything through that threat lens.

We've mentioned workplace supports in the previous section. Making sure you have micro supports in place that connect you and help you get back to that more balanced worldview is an essential part of self-care. Micro supports at work might include caring interactions with colleagues, making use of the small generosities such as the water cooler, the free tea and coffee, the places set aside for breaks. Outside your workplace make sure you spend time with your social support groups, people who bring you joy and who allow you to be your authentic self. While these things might seem obvious, they are often the first things we ditch when we are stressed and pressed for time. It is important to reframe them, prioritise them as self-care and replenish your wellbeing.

## Setting Boundaries

Setting clear boundaries is another essential self-care practice, especially for people working with clients who have experienced trauma. While we know that setting boundaries is important and that boundaries take maintenance, you have to keep checking and reinforcing them. When you're out of balance, you have allowed one area of your life to encroach on another. For many First Nations Peoples, boundaries were about staying in balance: staying connected, showing respect and reciprocity, staying in the safety of belonging to Country, which is grounding. If you think of boundaries as spaces where we come to meet and share with others, moving that line further inside your space means that you share more than you want to. The experience of collective trauma from colonisation has violated those practices, principles and values on a number of different levels, pulling us away from that centre that makes us well. The SEWB Wheel can be seen as a compass to navigate our way towards a new balance (Schultz, 2020).

When you work with people who've experienced trauma, it's important to understand that their ability to hold their boundaries is different from those who don't have the same trauma story. This inability is particularly harmful if there has been abuse in early childhood. The child's boundaries became blurred, which influences the developing brain, changing the development of what that young person considers normal. This occurs not only because their boundaries may have been violated by a perpetrator, but also because responding from the *drive for connection* can outweigh the risk of breaking a boundary, even when it's damaging.

It's also important to remember that boundaries are culture-specific. There are cultural differences between what's considered okay and what's not okay. For example, in collective communities extended family members often have the same responsibilities as a primary caregiver. We discussed these differences when we explored attachment theory in Chap. 4.

To avoid vicarious trauma or burnout you need to make space to reground and give yourself safety away from the pressures of working with trauma, so your nervous system does get to rest. It takes energy to maintain those boundaries.

## Planning Time for You

Planning time for yourself is a whole of brain activity. If you plan something, you allocate time to do it. That strategising brain redirects the threat activation, bringing your whole brain to the party, which is important for building resilience. When you plan time for you and you don't keep to that plan, placing other people's needs before yours, ask yourself, "why am I abandoning my wellbeing?".

## Nurturing Your Spirit

Many people have strong reactions to the word 'spiritual growth' or 'spirit', yet we know it is foundational; we know it's what makes us who we are. While it has different meanings in different cultures, it's also different for every person. How you find spiritual peace, what you consider your spirit and how you support and grow that is a very individual thing. Whatever it is, attending to that part of your being is very beneficial.

## Sleeping or Resting?

Before we leave this section, we want to point out that sleep itself is not necessarily rest. Replenishing requires rest and revitalisation of all the elements that make you *you*, all the functioning parts of your body. While you're *sleeping*, your brain is busy putting short-term memory into long-term memory. While your muscles and other parts of your body are *resting*, your brain is washing itself. Sleep is critical, of course, but it does not always replenish. And in fact, 'binge sleeping' doesn't compensate you for accumulated sleep deprivation. You might want to check out the book

*Why We Sleep* (Walker, 2017) to learn more about what's happening in your body and brain while you sleep.[3]

**Activity 8.3 Reflections on Rest**

- How do you find space to rest your spirit?
- How do you make a sanctuary where your nervous system and your limbic system can be at peace?
- How do you find a space where your creative brain is able to explore and replenish itself?

## Concluding Comments

Self-care is also about neuroscience, it's about physically what's happening in your brain and your body and what needs to happen for you to actually take good care of yourself. If you like what you do, if you like the job you do and you like being of help and being of service, then take care of yourself because people need you. Look out for those warning signs of vicarious trauma and compassion fatigue. Look out for those things that you hear, from what you hear yourself saying and what you hear your colleagues saying. One question you can ask yourself when you are considering something to do for your own self-care is: "Does it bring me joy?" If it brings you joy, you're getting some feel-good hormone, you're getting some good chemical release.

Finally, what strikes us when we spend this time talking about compassion fatigue and self-care is how much it is based in a non-Indigenous perspective. It is so far out of balance, so based on an individualist understanding of the world. Everything we hear about self-care tends to be about protecting the individual. From a collective perspective, self-care is a more holistic concept. Rather than changing you, you may need to change the circumstances you are in. It doesn't make sense to keep the focus on repairing the individual when it is the environment that needs to be fixed. Perhaps part of your self-care is changing policy and practices in your workplace.

[3] Check out the websites of Indigenous Health Australia https://iaha.com.au/ and the Australian Association of Social Workers https://www.aasw.asn.au/ for more information on self-care when working with clients.

**Activity 8.4 Check out and Reflection**

Take some time now to listen to your body. What are you feeling? Where in your body do you feel it?

This has been a big and important topic, one that may have you thinking about and reflecting on your own experiences.

How would you answer the following questions?

- What were the most important ideas you will take away from this chapter?
- What experience have you had with vicarious trauma, vicarious PTSD, compassion fatigue or burnout?
- What do you do for self-care?
- What self-care strategies nurture your spirit or bring you joy?
- What strategies might be more like distractions?

## References and Further Reading

Adams, R. E., Boscarino, J. A., & Figley, C. R. (2006). Compassion fatigue and psychological distress among social workers: A validation study. *American Journal of Orthopsychiatry, 76*(1), 103–108.

Archibald, J. (2008). *Indigenous storywork: Educating the heart, mind, body, and spirit*. UBC Press.

Bandura, A. (1997). *Self-efficacy: The exercise of control*. W.H. Freeman.

Coddington, K. (2017). Contagious trauma: Reframing the spatial mobility of trauma within advocacy work. *Emotion, Space and Society, 24*, 66–73.

Dalton-Smith, S. (2018). *Sacred rest: Recover your life, renew your energy, restore your sanity*. FaithWords.

Eades, A.-M., Hackett, M., Raven, M., Liu, H., & Cass, A. (2020). The impact of Vicarious Trauma on Indigenous health researchers. *Public Health Research and Practice*. Retrieved from https://doi.org/10.17061/phrp30012000

Foa, E. B., & Kozak, M. J. (1986). Emotional processing of fear: Exposure to corrective information. *Psychological Bulletin, 99*(1), 20–35. https://doi.org/10.1037/0033-2909.99.1.20

Figley, C. R. (1995). *Compassion fatigue: Coping with secondary traumatic stress disorder in those who treat the traumatized*. Brunner-Routledge.

Frankcom, K., Stevens, B., & Watts, P. (2016). *Fit to practice: Everything you wanted to know about starting your own psychology practice in Australia but were afraid to ask*. Australian Academic Press.

Grand, D. (2013). *Brainspotting: The revolutionary therapy for rapid and effective change*. Sounds True.

Hassing, C., & Quayle, C. (2019). Trauma informed practice: Working with communities affected by intergenerational trauma and managing vicarious trauma. *Native Title Newsletter, 1*, 15–17.

McCann, L. I., & Pearlman, L. A. (1990). Vicarious traumatization: A framework for understanding the psychological effects of working with victims. *Journal of traumatic stress, 3*(1), 131–149. https://doi.org/10.1002/jts.2490030110

McGrath, L., & Reavey, P. (2016). "Zip me up, and cool me down": Molar narratives and molecular intensities in 'helicopter' mental health services. *Health & Place, 38*, 61–69. https://doi.org/10.1016/j.healthplace.2015.12.005

Munari, S. C., Wilson, A. N., Blow, N. J., Homer, C. S. E., & Ward, J. E. (2021). Rethinking the use of 'vulnerable'. *Australian and New Zealand Journal of Public Health, 45*(3), 197–199.

Parker, G., Tavella, G., & Eyers, K. (2021). *Burnout: A guide to identifying burnout and pathways to recovery*. Allen & Unwin.

Pearlman, L., & Caringi, J. (2009). Living and working self-reflectively to address vicarious trauma. In C. A. Courtois & J. D. Ford (Eds.), *Treating complex traumatic stress disorders: Scientific foundations and therapeutic models* (pp. 202–222). The Guildford Press.

Rauvola, R. S., Vega, D. M., & Lavigne, K. N. (2019). Compassion fatigue, secondary traumatic stress, and vicarious traumatization: A qualitative review and research agenda. *Occupational Health Science, 3*(3), 297–336. https://doi.org/10.1007/s41542-019-00045-1

Reuben. (2015). When PTSD is contagious. *The Atlantic*. Retrieved from https://www.theatlantic.com/health/archive/2015/12/ptsd-secondary-trauma/420282/

Roche, A. M., Duraisingam, V., Trifonoff, A., Battams, S., Freeman, T., Tovell, A., Weetra, D., & Bates, N. (2013). Sharing stories: Indigenous alcohol and other drug workers' well-being, stress and burnout. *Drug and Alcohol Review, 32*(5), 527–535. https://doi.org/10.1111/dar.12053

Leiter, M. P. (2018). Burnout as a developmental process: Consideration of models. In W. Schaufeli, C. Maslach, & T. Marek (Eds.), *Professional Burnout: Recent developments in theory and research* (pp. 237–250). Taylor & Francis.

Schultz, C. (2020). *Factors of holistic wellbeing for members of the Aboriginal health and community workforce.* (PhD), Griffith University, Brisbane.

Shapiro, R., & Brown, L. S. (2019). Eye movement desensitization and reprocessing therapy and related treatments for trauma: An innovative, integrative trauma treatment. *Practice Innovations, 4*(3), 139–155.

Sodeke-Gregson, E. A., Holttum, S., & Billings, J. (2013). Compassion satisfaction, burnout, and secondary traumatic stress in UK therapists who work with adult trauma clients. *European Journal of Psychotraumatology, 4*(1), 21869. https://doi.org/10.3402/ejpt.v4i0.21869

Sprang, G., Clark, J. J., & Whitt-Woosley, A. (2007). Compassion fatigue, compassion satisfaction, and burnout: Factors impacting a professional's quality of life. *Journal of Loss and Trauma, 12*(3), 259–280. https://doi.org/10.1080/15325020701238093

Stamm, B. H. (2002). Measuring compassion satisfaction as well as fatigue: Developmental history of the compassion satisfaction and fatigue test. In C. R. Figley (Ed.), *Treating compassion fatigue* (Vol. 1, pp. 107–119). Brunner-Routledge.

Walker, M. (2017). *Why we sleep: Unlocking the power of sleep and dreams*. Scribner.

# 9

# Billabong of Culture and Healing

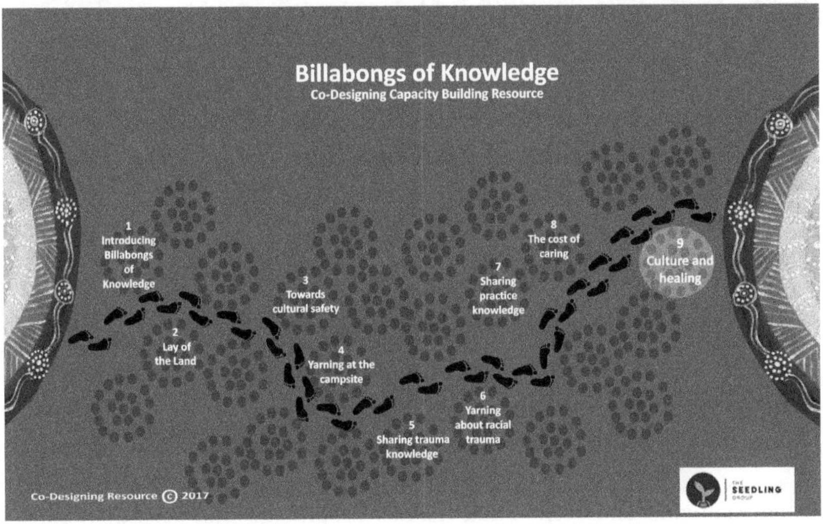


We acknowledge the traditional custodians of the land on which I write today, and the traditional custodians of the land on which you are reading this in my future. We pay our respects to Elders past, present and emerging and to their connection to the sea and waterways, the land and sky; strong in culture which endures from before, and despite of, the imposition of concrete, bitumen, foreign laws, and meritocracy. We thank them for reminding us that we have our own ways of knowing, being and doing.

**Riley O'Connor-Horrill** Kabi Kabi and Australian South Sea Islander Speech Pathologist


N. Tujague, K. Ryan, *Cultural Safety in Trauma-Informed Practice from a First Nations Perspective*, https://doi.org/10.1007/978-3-031-13138-7_9

## Introduction

At this, the final billabong along our journey, we yarn about the role culture plays in healing. This yarning session takes a little bit of a winding road, like all yarns do. This is a story that moves away from the trauma story towards the story of healing and culture, the story from the viewpoint of First Nations Peoples. We look at the psychology of culture and what *healing*-informed practice (different from *trauma*-informed practice) looks like. We discuss why this is important, and how and why we privilege Indigenous knowledges and Indigenous voices. We talk about how we connect the pieces of culture that were impacted by colonisation. We offer examples of cultural practices and approaches that are practiced in Aboriginal and Torres Strait Islander cultures.

## Culture and Identity

These are big concepts. Every Aboriginal and Torres Strait Islander person you talk to about culture and identity will come up with different perspectives. Former Aboriginal and Torres Strait Islander Social Justice Commissioner Mick Gooda, says the following about cultural identity:

> For Aboriginal and Torres Strait Islander Peoples it is our beliefs, our culture, and our family histories that contribute to our sense of who we are and what we mean to others. They are our source of belonging—and they anchor us and steer our course through our lives (Gooda, 2011).

**Activity 9.1 Check-in**

This body scan picture (Fig. 9.1) from the research we talked about in Chap. 2 may help you check in with a specific feeling and where it might be located in your body. With all of this new knowledge about the nervous system and trauma, how are you seeing emotions now?

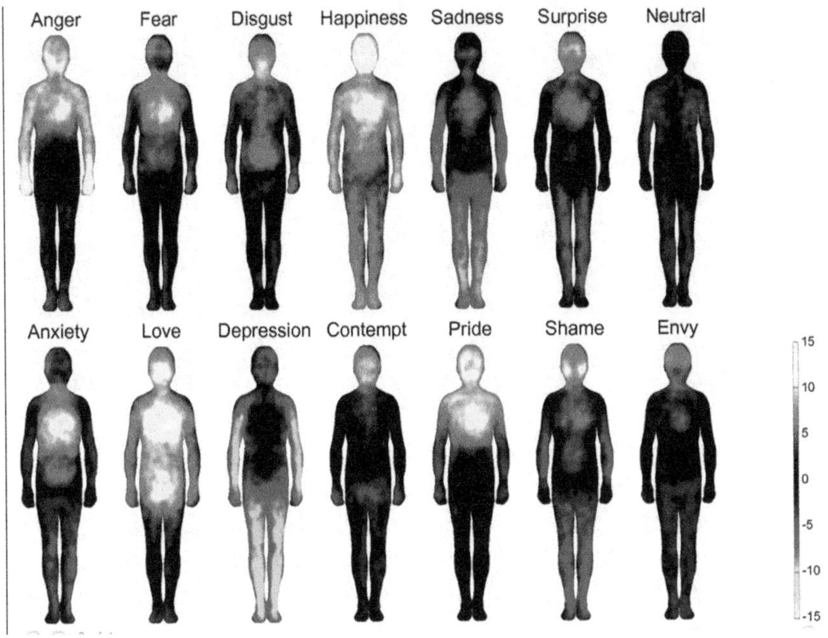


**Fig. 9.1** Emotions in the body

The elusive nature of how to describe 'culture' was beautifully put by a Torres Strait Islander man, who when asked the question 'what is culture', replied, "how can you ask me what culture is? Culture is the wind, the air; culture is the sand on my feet". That was him *feeling* culture, not defining culture by other people's words.

We also like Michael B. Salzman's idea of culture being a 'roadmap', which he outlines in his book, *A Psychology of Culture* (2018). He describes culture as something we grow up with that gives us all of our rules, all of our understanding, what is right, what is wrong.

## A Story of Culture and Identity

***Nicole:*** *I want to tell you a story about a young man I heard speak at a conference in Aotearoa (New Zealand). It was a life-changing moment for me. A young Māori man got up to speak and started telling his story. He stood in* *front of a big whiteboard. He had a marker pen in his hand. He went right up to the top right-hand corner of the whiteboard and drew something very small. He said this was the first canoe to come to Aotearoa. With my teacher hat on, I remember thinking, "why is he writing on the top right-hand corner of that whiteboard when there's this massive space to draw on?" Then he started to talk about the first people who came on that first canoe, and who their children were. He told us all their names, long, traditional Māori names.*

*Then he talked a little bit about the character of a particular person, and what their sister was like, what their brother was like, when they had children, who their children were. He just went on this long storytelling journey, literally filling up the whole of the whiteboard with all of these families and names and stories about people along the way. It was full of so much rich information. When he got right down to the bottom of the whiteboard he paused and said, "And then, he had a son. His name was Marcus. And that is me." I thought, like everybody in the room, "Oh my God. That is Marcus. That is him." This man could name all his ancestors from the people on the first canoe that came to Aotearoa, every single person in his family tree, in his culture, and what their stories were.*

*It really made me reflect on how our cultural lineage was interrupted by colonisation, particularly for so many people from the Stolen Generations in Australia. Even though we know our own family fairly well, I left that conference thinking, "I just want to go back and fill in all the gaps in our family tree." This powerful cultural introduction spoke really strongly to me about what culture is. It's about knowing who you are. Marcus understood the depth of the connectedness and obligation of each generation.*

## Symbiotic Relationships

Marcus went on to talk about symbiotic relationships. He does a lot of work with youth and said that the worst thing we can do for our young people is put them into institutional care. He said in a collective society we're meant to be surrounded by all of the symbiotic relationships that keep us thriving. He used the metaphor of the rainforest compared to the

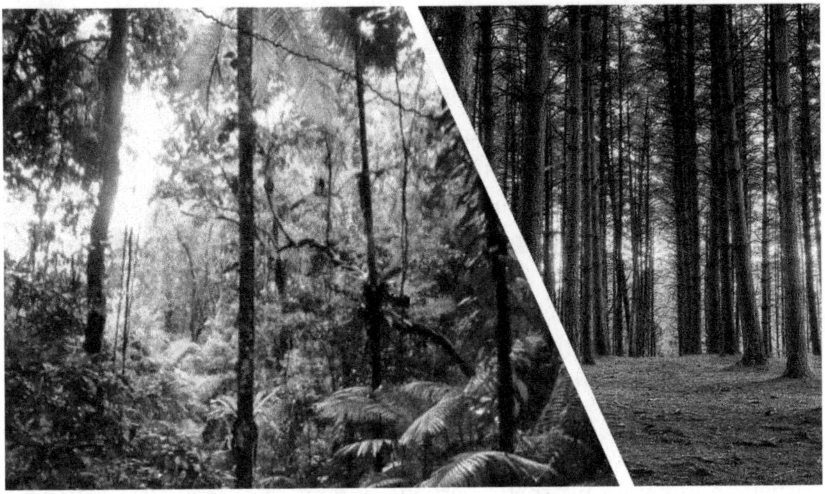

**Fig. 9.2** Symbiotic relationships. Source: Adapted from unsplash.com (open access)

pine forest (Fig. 9.2). In a rainforest there'll be mosses that can't survive with any sunlight on them. They'll be surviving nicely on the floor of the rainforest in the shade. There are the little ferns that can only have a sprinkling of light and are positioned just under the bigger ferns. That continues all the way up to the big trees that need full sunlight. All of those trees, bushes, ferns and mosses live in a symbiotic relationship with each other. As a collective community, we are like that. We need all of those symbiotic relationships around us.

When we're taken out of that community and put into an environment like a pine forest, where there's no diversity and no symbiotic relationships, it's just all the same. Pine forests are like institutions; they are places where it's not possible for our young people to thrive and be healthy. If you think of the developing brain and the connections that neurological development makes when it's coming across all these different stimuli, taking on all these messages and new relationships, growing all of those networks, you can understand why symbiotic relationships are so important for your development (see for example, Arnold et al., 2021).

## How Culture Heals

For many Indigenous peoples significant emotionally-activated events were followed by rituals, ceremony or celebration. For example, traditionally, after a war, a difficult journey or disasters and challenge, Aboriginal people would come together to rest and recover. This was often followed by ceremony of dance, song, giving thanks, grieving or wailing. There would be storytelling for men and women, teaching the young ones of the challenges and celebrating both the blessings and lessons learnt. This was all about returning to balance. This *replenishment* of mind, body and spirit is the 5th R in trauma-informed-care that we talk about in Chap. 8.

Western science now understands the benefits of returning your sympathetic and parasympathetic nervous systems to homeostasis as beneficial in minimising the cost of exposure to trauma. Scientists understand the importance of the connection of mind and body during times of traumatic stress and the importance of the return to normal biophysical and psychological states (Herman, 2015; Levine, 2010; Siegel, 2012; Van Der Kolk, 2015).

For Indigenous peoples and collective cultures of the world, this environment of safety occurs not in *being alone*, but in *being with oneself* within the collective community. The connection to the collective identity, culture, storylines, kinship and safety of belonging can be the beginning of healing. It builds upon resilience and the efficacy of the individual, the group and the collective.

### Water Music

This short video[1] is of women's water music (Fig. 9.3). Our great grandfather came from the island of Gaua in Vanuatu where women are famous for this cultural practice. They have been all over the world performing their water music. We had a go at learning how to do this water music, which is quite a process in itself! They make it look so easy.

[1] https://www.instagram.com/p/Bt6gtrYnWtp/?igshid=pjtgpwpnq6mf

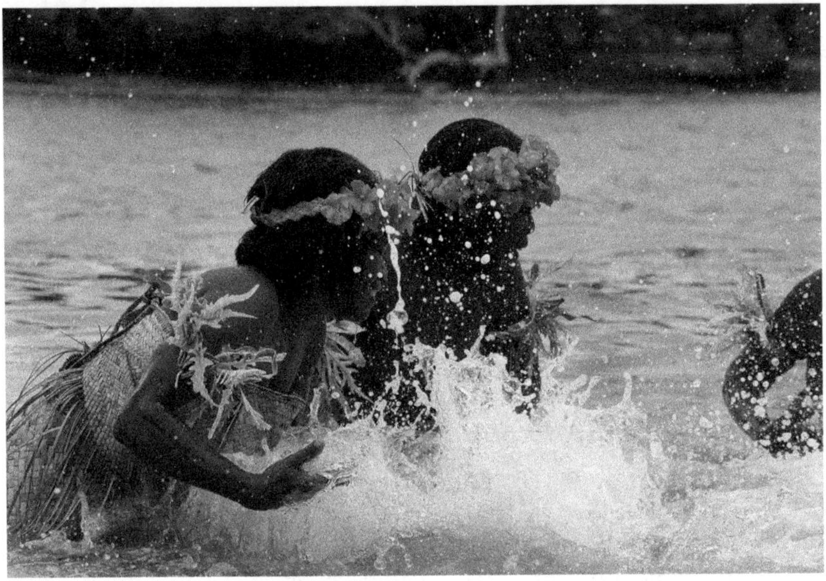

**Fig. 9.3** Water music women Gaua Island Vanuatu

***Kelleigh***: *When I first saw them, it just looked like they were having a whole lot of fun. They were splashing in the water and laughing and what's not fun about that? But then I realised there was a whole lot of other things going on. They were actually playing music, playing sounds, like songs, but they were water songs. And the unity we see there is really strong and beautiful.*

**Activity 9.2 Reflective questions on video**

Reflect on these questions when you're watching this clip:

- With everything we know about trauma, the brain and the body, what are three things you can see happening?
- What does this have to do with *your* story? What is important for you to understand while you watch this?
- What are two things that occur to you that could help you in your work?

***Nicole**: One thing I remember when I first watched it was that everybody had a part to play and they were all synchronised, part of one collective experience. They are held in high esteem by their communities and when it was time for them to begin, everybody cleared a path. Theirs is an important role in the community. I saw Elder status, women's business and knowledge-holding. I also saw storytelling, traditions being handed down, language and identity. Another important thing about this clip is that the women are dispersing stress chemicals from their bodies. They are producing feel-good chemicals. They are also one with Country. They're saltwater people and they're performing ceremony together in the salt water.*

## Rituals, Dance, Story and Songlines

The water music ceremony is a clear example of how culture can be healing. For generations, we as Aboriginal and Torres Strait Islander Peoples have had many different rituals that have served us well to keep us grounded and healthy. Mainstream Australia tends to see rituals and cultural artefacts as a static snippet of what happened a long time ago. But in fact, culture is ongoing and renewing itself all the time.

In the book *Sand Talk*, Aboriginal man Tyson Yunkaporta (2019) describes rituals, ceremony and dance stories as being the physical manifestation of what our ancestors are telling us about stories from the past, about our Dreaming, our beginning of time. Yunkaporta sees all of our rituals and ceremonies as metaphors: taking problem-solving messages and storylines and putting them into physical form. In this way they are a constant living part of our culture. Complex marriage lines, trading lines and ways of being were held in songlines.

> Everything starts and ends with Country in the Aboriginal worldview. Yet there are no endings in this worldview, nor are there any beginnings. Time and place are infinite and everywhere. Everything is part of a continuum, an endless flow of life and ideas emanating from Country, which some refer to as thc Dreaming.

> In the Dreaming, as in Country, there is no separation between the animate and inanimate. Everything is living—people, animals, plants, water and air. We speak of Sea, Land and Sky Country. Creator ancestors created the Country and its interface, the Dreaming. In turn, Dreaming speaks for Country. Country has Dreaming, Country is Dreaming … Songlines, related to Dreamings or Dreaming tracks, connect sites of knowledge embodied in the features of the land. It is along these routes that people travelled to learn from Country (Neale & Kelly, 2020, p. 1).

While this might be a hard concept to grasp, it's critically important. If you think of rituals in terms of retelling a story, in many ways what's happening is not only activating different systems in the brain, but also in the way it attaches to other stories, to meaning-making, to caring for land and caring for family.

Yunkaporta also talks about creation in relation to what happens when you hear a joke. When you hear something that's funny, which is usually something you haven't made that connection with before, like gazelles talking to lions, he says that the endorphin hit you get is so strong, it actually makes you spontaneously laugh out loud. Hearing a joke creates a new neural network. It's all part of creation, which is ongoing. That's a refreshing way to think about creation, not about 'where it all started', but as an ongoing story. We know our culture, our stories, our beliefs and that's the cultural roadmap that guides us.

## Weaving as a Protective Factor

This picture of an Indigenous woman weaving (Fig. 9.4) is another example of how culture protects, how healing happens holistically. She went out as part of a group to collect and prepare the palm leaves. There would be a recipe in her weaving that's been handed down, a pattern that belongs to her family group. This tells her who she is. This is part of her identity. The very fact that she can recreate that pattern, builds her self-esteem. She's sitting on Country. We now know more about what happens in the body when you sit on Country (Jones et al., 2018). In mainstream terms we think of healing and wellness as a scientific biomedical thing, but

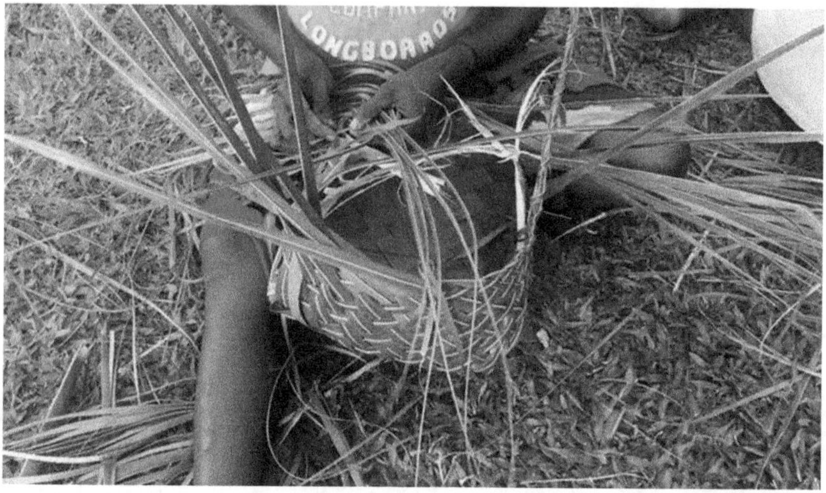


**Fig. 9.4** Weaving on Gaua Island Vanuatu. Photo taken by Nicole Tujague

these cultural practices heal in a more holistic way. They continue to be part of the survival mechanism of peoples who have lived in collective cultures over many generations.

***Kelleigh***: *A Torres Strait Islander man once said to me that their woven mats are a symbol of life. You are born on a mat, you live your life on a mat, and when you die you were buried in a mat. You come into this world and leave this world on a mat.*

## Culture in Self-Care

Western culture silos all the different activities of self-care. We know exercise is good for you, eating well is good for you, singing and dancing are good for you, getting enough rest is good for you. While there are benefits from each of these activities, without meaning they are just chores, just another thing you have to do for your health; they don't deliver well-being. When you think about the SEWB Wheel, what's missing is connection in these individual activities. What you do culturally that embodies physical movement and connection, like fishing or hunting or dance or ceremony, is replenishing in a holistic way. They are not just empty physical movements. It's about incorporating culture into your physical activity in a way that creates connection and embeds meaning that supports holistic wellbeing rather than separating body from spirit.

Traditionally, song, dance, ceremony and storytelling were connected to culture, meaning and identity (Guerin et al., 2011). The meaning is the connection, which is what was severed by colonisation and siloing of elements of culture and activity. Replenishing that connection is replenishing wellbeing. Explaining what meaning really is, what connection really is, is about conveying the beauty within the sacred properties of language, songs, dances and designs that are owned in perpetuity and deployed in ceremony by specific groups within cultures, within Aboriginal and Torres Strait Islander groups. These rights function as 'title deeds' ancestrally-bestowed interests in specific lands, seas, homelands (Corn & Gumbula, 2021).

First Nations Peoples' ceremonies and rituals continue to hold meaning, for the benefit of both the individual and the collective. The knowledge behind these practices is underpinned by a deep understanding of the importance of physical activity for the wellbeing of body and spirit. Practising self-awareness is another example; it is essential for grounding. It allows us to activate our limbic system fully and engage the frontal cortex so we can make sense of what's happening when we are triggered (Lou et al., 2017).

***Kelleigh***: *When I attended the first Aboriginal and Torres Strait Islander conference on suicide prevention held in Australia, there was a time when Aboriginal women left the conference to go outside. They stood barefoot and sat in the dry riverbed to ground themselves and connect back to their ancestors. This was the riverbed where their ancestors had camped and slept. Each drew strength to be present in the work for the collective. Overall, it was that absolute understanding of the importance of balance.*

Doing ceremonial dances, playing sport, all those things that move your major muscle groups, help to disperse the neurochemicals that the threat response produces, as we talked about in Chap. 4. When you're laughing, experiencing pleasure, comfort or relaxing, think of the context. You feel safe, you're with your 'tribe'. You are disengaging from the threat response. Laughing and pleasure lower your blood pressure, as it does when you cry, quicker than any drug can. There's good evidence that laughing increases dopamine and decreases cortisol, as do singing and dancing (Kreutz et al., 2012).

We all know that it's healthy to eat what's in season and what's grown locally. We've heard people say that when they are on Country and eating the traditional foods of that Country, they feel better. This is no surprise and is supported by research about Japan that shows if you're Japanese, you actually have the enzymes that it takes to digest soy products present in a traditional cultural diet, such as tofu, better than people who aren't of that culture (Enders, 2017). Consider finding out more about the health and medicinal properties of foods from your traditional lands.

***Nicole:*** *I remember working with some young girls who came from the Tiwi Islands. It was my job to look after them while they were at boarding school a long way from their home. I had a finite budget to take them out a couple of nights a month. When I'd say, "what do you guys want to eat?" they'd say, "We want barramundi. We want barramundi." And I'd think, "okay, there goes my budget." But we'd go out and we'd eat barramundi ('barra') at a local restaurant. They'd take a few bites and say, "oh, this is terrible." The barramundi was completely different from the barra they ate on their own lands. I noticed that the longer they were at boarding school, their skins got greyer and greyer. They became more unwell. When they'd come back from their home after school holidays, their skin would be glowing.*

## Privileging Aboriginal and Torres Strait Islander Knowledge Systems

If you have come to appreciate the healing capacity of culture, then you understand why it is important to prioritise Indigenous voices. This means talking with Indigenous people about what is important to know, what cultural practices are meaningful and contribute to healing. As Aboriginal and Torres Strait Islander Peoples, we were not just surviving on this continent before colonisation, we were thriving. We had a rich understanding of health and wellbeing. The Western world is adopting more and more pieces of Indigenous knowledge, sometimes without context. There is this incredible opportunity to learn from Indigenous Peoples by privileging and respecting those knowledge systems.

This becomes important when we start to think about how we evaluate Indigenous specific health programs in Australia. Too often when we evaluate programs from a non-Indigenous perspective; the questions that get asked are things like, "Was the program completed within budget? Was it completed on time? Were there enough participants to make the program valid? Did the program have the desired health or social outcomes? And if it didn't, what went wrong?". These questions only measure healing from one perspective. They are not necessarily the questions Indigenous Peoples, especially survivors of the Stolen Generations, want answered in order to measure a program's success.

***Nicole:*** *In my research with the men from the Kinchela Boys Home, whom we talk about in Chapter 5, the men are really clear that what should be measured is what healing means for them. Did it put together any of the pieces that were taken apart with colonisation? Does it go some way towards interrupting intergenerational trauma?*

This is another example of how two completely different knowledge systems focus on different priorities, informed by different values and worldviews. On the one hand, the non-Indigenous biomedical model focuses on symptoms and pathologies and tracing their origins, seeing healing in terms of getting rid of symptoms rather than investigating the holistic underlying causes. On the other hand, an Indigenous knowledge system considers the connection of all things and that the need for healing comes from the disruption caused by colonisation.

Pre-colonisation, Aboriginal and Torres Strait Islander Peoples thrived on this continent in a way that privileged relationships to Country. Living closely with Country has allowed Aboriginal and Torres Strait Islander Peoples to participate respectfully in the complexity of nature. Complexity theory (Berkes et al., 2008) goes some way to understanding how nature works with its many complex and interrelated systems. Having categorised every species and element, separating and breaking everything into its tiniest components, Western science is now continually delighted and sometimes horrified to 'discover' the infinite symbiotic relationships and systems that exist in every aspect of this planet (Redvers, et al., 2020).

For those who have always lived on this continent, there has always been the understanding that the world is a complex place of interdependent symbiotic relationships. We have passed on our understanding without reduction or simplification; this is seen as our cultural heritage. Our ways of living and our beliefs have grown out of nurturing our relationship with Country, manifesting in sophisticated systems to make sustainable what we take and give back. Take for example the fish trap,[2] a rock structure that traps fish when the tide goes out. To the coloniser, this may have looked like a way of harvesting meagre catches. In fact, it was taking just enough, and ensured fish stocks weren't fished out. What colonisers saw as primitive survival techniques, are now being recognised as sophisticated acts of sustainability (Pascoe, 2014).

In the modern world, societies are struggling with the implications of over consumption. They sometimes look to Indigenous cultures for sustainable practices but cannot resist cherry picking techniques and taking them in isolation, removing those practices from the complex system in which they belong. One example of this in Australia is the interest in traditional Aboriginal methods of fire management, known as cultural burning or 'fire-stick farming' (Bird et al., 2008). Those methods are often still interpreted through a non-Indigenous lens, which misses the holistic concept of why those rituals and practices work.

***Kelleigh**: This story demonstrates the lack of understanding of holistic approaches. This happened when Indigenous rangers and Elders were asked to teach cultural burning techniques. When non-Indigenous rangers started using the Indigenous burning practices in other places, they saw it is a way of back burning, without understanding the many specific things appropriate when using the techniques in different places. These contextual considerations mean that cultural burning is different everywhere. The non-Indigenous rangers went back to the Elders and said "we did what you told us to do, but it didn't work", the Elders said, "you did what you asked us about, but you have to let nature work with you, and understand the ecosystems, soil types, grasses as well as the type of ashes that will be left behind, in the different places you are burning". That was a hard lesson about contextual versus linear understandings, about asking for answers rather than looking for meaning.*

[2] Visit https://aiatsis.gov.au/brief-introduction-indigenous-fishing to see examples of fish traps.

*It's still privileging one knowledge system and borrowing a bit from another or fitting the other within the dominant system, which is not necessarily going to work.*

## Respecting Aboriginal and Torres Strait Islander Cultural Strengths

Aboriginal and Torres Strait Islander Peoples see the past as part of the present and future, all as one. It is all part of who we are. It is all interconnected (Neale & Kelly, 2020). Mainstream memory, especially in Australia, tends to see the past as over and done with; it enjoys the benefits and tends to take little responsibility for what has been done to our people, to our cultures. While we as First Nations Peoples are *required* to walk in both worlds, non-Indigenous people can't walk in ours. While reconciliation involves everyone, it can only be achieved when it's Indigenous-led.

For many First Nations Peoples, cultural rules provide a map for our lives. We are related and responsible for our Country, songs, storylines, birds, animals, trees, mountains, waterways. These are all connected in memory through songlines. The past, the present and future are nonlinear, they are all interrelated (Neale & Kelly, 2020). We have a complex system of *reciprocal responsibility*.

In her book of essays, *These Precious Days*, Ann Patchett (2021), talks about a friend who trains forest rangers. Her friend always starts by asking her students: "do you love nature?" to which they all reply "yes". She then asks: "do you believe that nature loves you?" They're confused by this question. Maybe at its heart, this is the difference between Indigenous and non-Indigenous thinking. For Indigenous Peoples, the reciprocal relationship is clear; the answer is "yes".

When you as an individual know you are responsible for and are part of that bigger system, it allows you to know your place in the world, and in knowing your place in the world, you come to know your identity. The more you know your identity, the more you understand who you are and how to live a life that is true to that identity.

Another important thing we know when we are able to practise culture is its potent *protective effect*. It develops our resilience. While we all have different traumas that happen through our lifetimes, a strong culture and identity can protect us (Guerin et al., 2011). Communities that have continued the practice of culture can govern themselves based on their rules; they can speak their languages; they fare so much better. This type of 'cultural continuity' becomes a potent protective factor (Chandler & Lalonde, 1998, 2008).

***Kelleigh:*** A *Western Desert woman once told me, "we look after our children until it is time for them to look after us". That's why when we break up family systems, traditional family ways of being are disrupted.*

## Connection to Country

***Nicole:*** *The real meaning of connection to Country is very hard to explain to people who think within a non-Indigenous knowledge system. I've sat in lectures with visiting Indigenous lecturers and asked them, "tell us a little bit about connection to Country. What does it mean for you?" A man from the Yuin Nation said, "it's the feeling I get when I drive up the road and into my Country. It's what I can smell and what I can feel". The answers are always diverse. For me, it's like my body on a cellular level recognises everything in a different way when I'm on my own Country. The air is different. The sounds are different. My senses are picking up something that tells me I'm on Country. Understanding what connection to Country is has far reaching implications. We've had anthropologists ring us and say, "We need to understand. We're doing this Native Title work and we need to understand this connection to land."*

Yunkaporta (2019) talks about this connection in a beautiful way. He uses the metaphor of a woven basket in a flowing stream. The water as it flows through the basket is like our life or our creation, it's never static. It's always creating something different. He talks about how who we are is not just based in our physical bodies, but our artefacts and our land can also become part of us. For instance, if you're using a pen to write something, part of who you are is going into that pen and going onto that page. Suddenly, you're not just you, you're the words that you're writing. Sometimes, you won't think about what you've written until you pick up that pen. The pen itself connects you back with that knowledge. That knowledge is not just being in you, it's connected to all the things that you come in contact with, the things you make, the conversations you have with people. If I have a conversation with you about something interesting or important to both of us, it might be that in two years' time when I see you again, that knowledge comes back with that relationship. Our connection to land is like that. Part of us connects to our Country. That's why being removed from Country is so painful for Aboriginal and Torres Strait Islander Peoples, because it's disconnecting us from something that's part of us. What Yunkaporta does is get you thinking outside of that idea of just being this physical human body, to how our relationships and our connections to everything are part of who we are as well (Bawaka Country et al., 2014; Burgess et al., 2009).

## The Dreaming and Creation

This beautiful artwork by Bronwyn Haynes (Smith) is one we purchased for a project we worked on, depicting the Rainbow Serpent (Fig. 9.5), one of the Aboriginal creation stories. Like the idea of creation, the Dreaming is a concept that has had a non-Indigenous lens put over it and

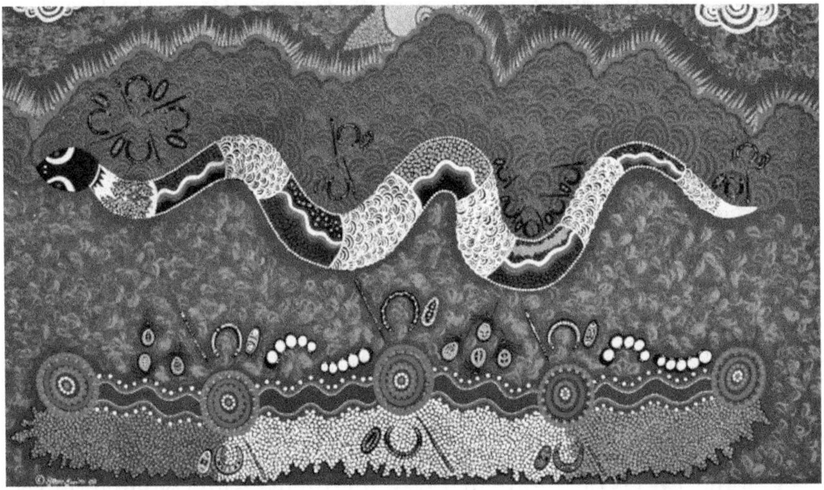

**Fig. 9.5** Story Telling after the Gathering of Bush Tucker. Source: Artist Bronwyn Haynes (Smith)

is largely misunderstood. Every different clan has its own story about their Dreaming. It's not this thing that happened a long time ago; it's part of an evolving living culture. Tyson Yunkaporta tells a creation story associated with the constellation of Orion:

> … a Big Bang caused by Echidna fighting with Turtle. The trauma of this event caused the sky camp and earth camp to separate, and the universe to begin deep cycles of expansion and contraction, like breathing, in a pattern shaping everything.
>
> The Big Bang pattern, that initial point of impact, is not just something that occurs at the massive scale of the universe but is repeated infinitely in all its lands and parts. Many creation stories refer to this point of impact, often represented by a stone at the centre of the place and story. Uluru is the stone at the centre of this continent's story, a pattern repeated in the interconnected and diverse stories of many smaller regions, reflected in our own bodies at the navel and then down into smaller and smaller parts at the quantum level of our cosmology. In this way of knowing, there is no difference between you, a stone, a tree or a traffic light. All contain knowledge, story, pattern (Yunkaporta, 2019, pp. 28–29).

These stories not only give you meaning and language, but connection to place. Your totems are born from that connection and those stories. Totems acknowledge the equal existence of other creatures we live with and define our role within the group. It's a relationship between natural entities, persons and groups. This is so all creatures and humans can live in harmony. The creation stories form your morality and values that underpin your culture (Kwaymullina, 2005). It is a worldview where humans are part of nature, not distinct from other creatures, sharing with them the same life essence. It's a relationship between a person or a group of persons and a natural object or animal as part of nature.

## Language and Culture

One of the aspects of culture that was interrupted with colonisation was language. Language is such an important part of our culture, who we are and our identity.

***Nicole**: Sometimes I try to imagine what it would be like if everybody in France suddenly wasn't allowed to speak French anymore. Language holds so much more than the literal translation. I remember when I was in France once and I told my mother-in-law that I was going to go window shopping and she said: "oh, you're going lèche-vitrines." I said, "Oh, is that window shopping in French?" She said, "yes, it literally means 'licking the windows'". I thought that's such a great translation, something that really belongs to that language. Often meaning is carried in what is not said in languages or in what doesn't need to be said because of a shared knowing.*

As language is such an important part of who we are, when language was stripped from us, when people went to missions and children's homes and foster homes and weren't allowed to speak language any longer, they were left not only with big holes in their vocabulary, but they also lost a big part of their identity. It's estimated that prior to colonisation there were 250 distinct Aboriginal and Torres Strait Islander languages and about 600 dialects.[3] A hundred different languages exist in some form now in Australia, but many of those languages are at risk of becoming extinct (Hobson et al., 2010). Cultural concepts and knowledge are also carried through language. When you lose your language, you lose an important part of your cultural knowledge and the true original meaning of those cultural concepts.

There are programs in Australia that aim to restore Aboriginal and Torres Strait Islander languages (Hobson et al., 2010). When bilingual education programs were established in the Northern Territory and Western Australia, kids started learning things at school in their own language, which made a huge impact as suddenly they were connecting with the content and understanding what they were supposed to be learning. It starts with understanding how critical language is to identity. It's not something that's not needed because now we've all got English. It's so much more than just translating what you're thinking into words. It's part of who you are. Your whole cultural worldview is influenced by your language.

[3] See The Healing Foundation website https://healingfoundation.org.au/

## Dadirri and Yarning

There is much knowledge that First Nations cultures can share with non-Indigenous knowledge systems. Sharing knowledge is a type of reconciliation, which is healing in itself. An example is what Dr Miriam-Rose Ungunmerr-Baumann (2017) calls *dadirri*, that deep inner spring inside of us, that deep listening. It's one of the foundations of yarning circles (Barlo et al., 2020; Hughes & Barlo, 2020). When you sit in a yarning circle and practice *dadirri*, it's about listening to what the other person is saying without thinking, "what am I going to say next? Is that right or is that wrong?" or passing judgment. It's about listening respectfully, absorbing the words and their meanings, and deciding if you have anything meaningful to add to the conversation. It's about listening to learn, adding what's being said to your existing knowledge, not just listening to have input. You can't listen if your head is full of what you want to say. When it's your turn to share, there's a place for your knowledge, or *not*, if that's what you've learned by the time you get to speak! Remember the circle is about the collective, not about the individual.

Yarning in the non-Indigenous sense of the word can mean a range of things. It can just mean having a yack with someone over a cup of tea. In the Aboriginal sense, there are lots of different types of yarning and we're starting to use yarning a lot more now in the classroom and in meetings, and for research and collecting data (Bessarab & Ng'andu, 2010). One of the most important things yarning does is to mitigate the power imbalance in the room; you don't have someone controlling everything. Everybody has an opportunity to have a voice, say exactly what they think without fear of judgement. Participants practice *dadirri* while someone else is speaking. They are required to wait for their turn. If you have to wait until it's your turn to speak in the yarning circle, by the time you've heard everybody you have a much better understanding of what people are saying. You've heard other people properly. Quite often you end up saying something completely different from what all that clutter in your brain was trying to make you say. So, while *dadirri* and yarning are two cultural practices, they can be used in non-Indigenous contexts as gifts that help us work in a richer and more productive way.

If you're only listening to either validate or justify your own view, you are in that heightened arousal state. That will make it much harder to remember or fully understand what people in the circle are saying. You won't be growing knowledge or making meaning from what is being said in the circle. *Dadirri* and yarning drives understanding and connectedness (Crouch, 2017).

## Collective Healing

Healing from collective trauma takes a collective approach. This bus is a wonderful example, with its words: 'unlocking our past to free our future' (Fig. 9.6). What the KBHAC men have done is put together a program which takes their stories to the community. At the front of the bus, you'll see all the numbers given to the men when they arrived as small children to the Kinchela Boys' Home. The men take the bus into communities, into schools and tell people the stories about what it was like for them as kids. They tell their stories in a safe way, as safe as they can make it for the children.

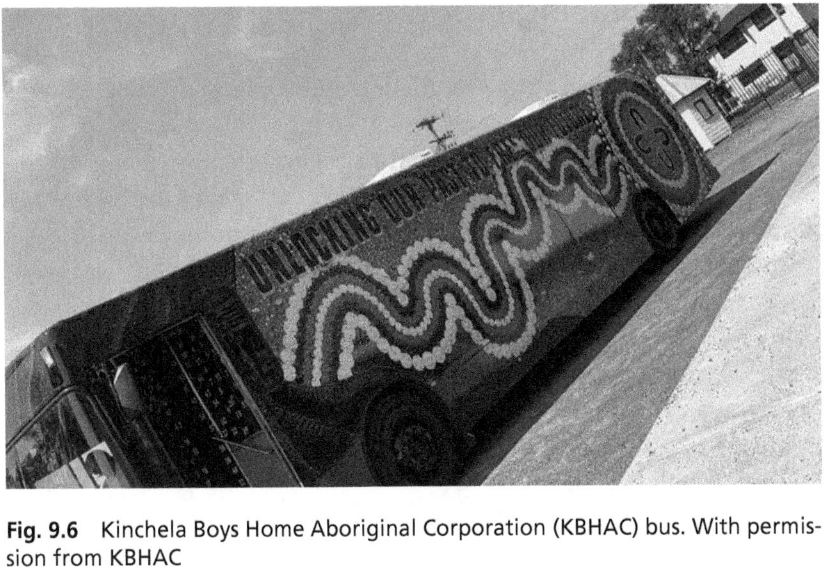


**Fig. 9.6** Kinchela Boys Home Aboriginal Corporation (KBHAC) bus. With permission from KBHAC

This is truth telling on a collective level, vital for healing trauma of this magnitude. The KBHAC men have come together and are now able to tell their truth; they're able to talk about what happened to them, many for the first time. They are still finding their families today through *Link-Up*,[4] which finds families who were broken up when their children were taken and reconnect them back to their Countries and their relatives. What we are now seeing is people at last finding out where they came from; people putting together those missing links; people rebuilding those relationships and those understandings. Sometimes those reunions are graveside reunions.

If you go to the Healing Foundation website[5] you'll hear members of the Stolen Generations telling their stories. One is from Aunty Faye who says, "we were told we weren't black" and then she says, "and we believed them." Despite being dark skinned, she says, "we used to walk on the other side of the road and look across the road and think we're not like them, *we're* not Aboriginal". Even though this brainwashing went on, in the interview Aunty Faye laughs about believing that. Being able to tell the story and see the humour is another sign of healing.

## Collective Healing Programs

As we discovered when we talked about cultural safety and racial trauma, working with individual clients through trauma-informed practice can be healing and very helpful for that one person. When we discussed collective trauma in Chap. 5, we talked about the impact of the breakdown of relationships with members of the Stolen Generations, the breakdown of cultural language and connections. Once we understand that, it is clear why collective healing might look different from what an individualist culture thinks of as healing. The Healing Foundation has developed this model (Fig. 9.7) based on a literature review drawn from First Nations programs across the world (Grealy et al., 2015). It identifies the elements that need to be present for collective healing to happen. We discuss in

[4] https://www.linkupnsw.org.au/

[5] https://healingfoundation.org.au/

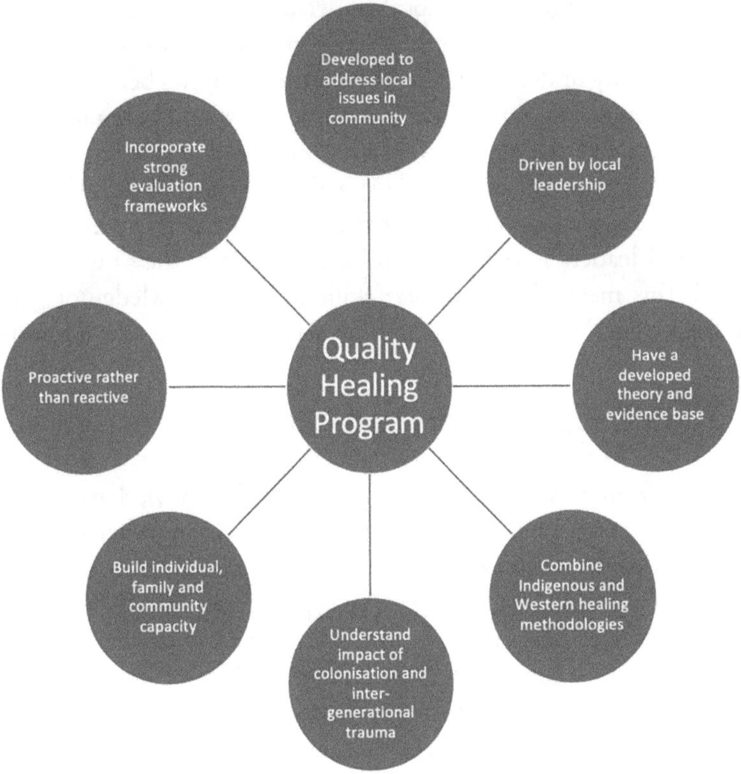


**Fig. 9.7** Elements of a quality healing program for Aboriginal and Torres Strait Islander Peoples. Source: Grealy et al. (2015, p. 11)

detail the elements that are most relevant for our purposes: local leadership, strong evidence base, proactive rather than reactive, and addressing local issues.

## Driven by Local Leadership

The Healing Foundation has done a lot of research into what contributes to effective healing for First Nations Peoples who have been affected by collective trauma around the world (The Healing Foundation, 2019; Blignault et al., 2014). One of the most important drivers of success in collective healing programs is local leadership. Nobody understands the worldview of community members like someone from within that community. Nobody understands the history, the dynamics between families, the covert things that go on in community and what's going to work for a community, like the members, particularly the Elders, of that community. While you might have professional expertise and knowledge, the Elders and community members are the experts of their own lives. Talking to the local leaders is critical to collective healing. They must lead the process. This means bringing *your* skills to *their* knowledge of what is right, and what's wrong, and what is needed in *their* local communities.

## Have a Developed Theory and Evidence Base

'Evidence' from a Western worldview is what we say we have when we prove that when you do the same thing a certain number of times it achieves the same outcome. We call that 'cause and effect', which is what we're aiming for so we can say, "this practice works". In the non-Indigenous system, it's based on all those rules around what research or what a theory-base looks like. If we look at the idea of 'evidence' from a cultural worldview, we might still get the same result, but without writing it down. Traditionally, we were not about writing things down. If what we did was successful, it got repeated, if it didn't, it either got changed or improved or it wasn't practised again.

What often happens in the current system is that the funders of programs that are supposed to help us say, "we'll fund this one, because we've got all this 'peer-reviewed' research evidence, but we won't fund that one, because we've only got *anecdotal* evidence, meaning we only have your word for it that it works or doesn't work". Here again is that clash of two worldviews, which highlights disrespect for cultural knowledge holders. As an Aboriginal and Torres Strait Islander person, I might say, "just because you have good evidence defined by your worldview, doesn't mean it's actually going to work for me. But what I know about what I do and what works for us or what heals us, I have a lot of evidence because our communities have a lot of lived experience".

## Proactive, Rather Than Reactive

Being proactive rather than reactive is one of the common denominators of a successful healing model that works in collective communities. Unlike the Northern Territory Intervention that we talk about in Chap. 6, which rushed in as a major reaction to stories of child sexual abuse in some communities, the programs that work are based on understanding the core strengths that make a community healthy. These include rich kinship networks, cultural lore and protocols, strong local governance structures, autonomy and self-determination and connection to storylines and songlines.

## Developed to Address Local Issues in Community

Addressing local issues specific to a particular community marries well with that element of working with local leadership. What's important to that community and its cultural worldview may be unimportant or unrecognised within the worldview of the non-Indigenous system that's trying to help. One example might be when there's not enough water in a particular community, the mainstream solution might be to bring in tanks or build a pipeline. Perhaps if they had listened to the locals, they may have learned about local springs that would have been more appropriate to attend to and put down wells there. Bringing in infrastructure that those communities may not be able to support or maintain (let alone fund), may not work for the local people, becoming an ongoing problem for them to deal with.

Another example is building houses that don't fit the climate or the way people live in communities. When the people don't use the houses in the way the non-Indigenous system intended them to, then the local people are labelled as 'negligent' or 'destructive' or 'not appreciative'. Who's that solution working for? Again, that is another way our people are pathologised because they weren't consulted or listened to. Working in a healing-informed way would include collaborating with people in community to meet their housing needs.

While much of our focus in this book so far has been on trauma-informed practice, many Indigenous organisations and researchers are moving beyond that now and are looking more into *healing*-informed practice (Grealy et al., 2015). While cultural safety in trauma-informed practice is foundational, think about how your practice could be more healing-focused, more healing-informed. How do you incorporate cultural healing and a knowledge system that may be different from your own into your practice? If you're an Aboriginal or Torres Strait Islander person, how do you give voice to your knowledge system, and embrace all the healing parts of that in everything you do in your life and in your work?

A good resource we recommend is the *Working Together* book edited by Pat Dudgeon, Helen Milroy and Roz Walker (2014) that we have mentioned in earlier chapters. A useful guide from that book is this model of pathways to recovery from transgenerational trauma or intergenerational trauma (Fig. 9.8):

The authors take three of the legacies of colonisation that devastated communities and look at ways to heal from the damage. Empowering communities with their own governance and their own decision-making is critically important to healing.

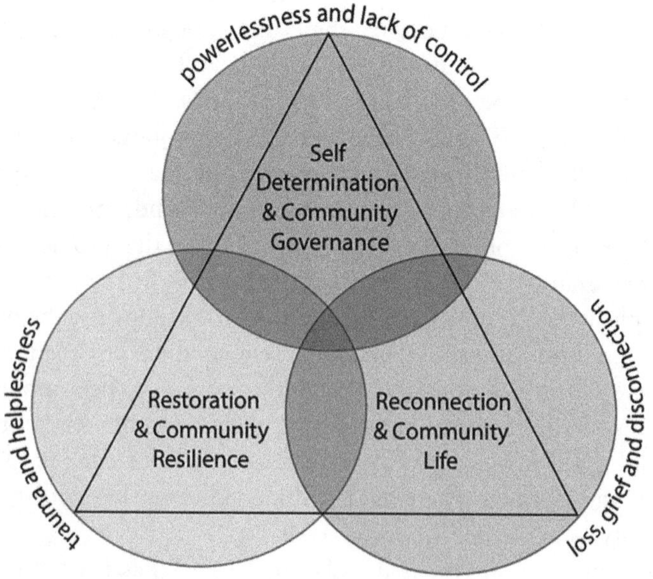


**Fig. 9.8** Pathways to recovery from transgenerational trauma. Source: Dudgeon, Milroy & Walker (2014, p. 424)

## Understanding Traditional Healing

The *Ngangkaṟi* traditional healers, who are Western Desert people in Central Australia (Ngaanyatjarra Pitjantjatjara Yankunytjatjara Women's Council Aboriginal Corporation, 2013), say when you're unwell, it's about where your Spirit is sitting in your body or if it's left your body. These healers see your Spirit, which inhabits your body and gives you your life force and how you navigate the world. Everything in bush medicine is about reconnecting and bringing that vibration back into balance.

The *Ngangkaṟi* say when people indulge in drugs and alcohol and promiscuous behaviour, their Spirit is lost and it's looking for somewhere to belong. They're looking for connection, often in the wrong places. When people experience vicarious trauma, they have this extra burden that carries them from their centre. For the young ones, they lose their connection to the *strength* of their cultural identity and take on this deficit model of being black, which cannot do anything but harm them. They lose the connection to the ways that keep them strong. Watch this beautiful video of *Ngangkaṟi* healers doing their work.[6]

***Kelleigh:*** *I've often heard people say, when they notice they're unwell, that they don't connect, they don't listen to Spirit talking to them; they no longer listen to their ancestors; they've stopped listening to their brother and sister animals; they've stopped listening to their body; they're all in their head; they're not connected; they forget who they are. Their Spirit is no longer keeping them grounded in the now. They are often angry or tired, and the reason is if you're not connected, you don't draw strength from, you don't share energy with, everything that surrounds you. Country can't replenish you and relationships can't replenish you, because you're not really there. You're all alone. People say to me "I don't feel right way".*

This video of Uncle Bob Randall explains it really well when he talks about the connection to land, spirit and Country for Aboriginal people.[7]

---

[6] https://www.youtube.com/watch?v=YyNlJdrZBPE&ab_channel=TheFeedSBS

[7] https://www.youtube.com/watch?v=xVhZwU2x9Jk&ab_channel=PortraitsinFaith

## Want to know more about cultural healing programs?

For untold millennia, First Nations Peoples across the world used healing practices that kept them well, spiritually, socially, physically and mentally. Since the recognition of the direct relationship between the impact of historical and intergenerational trauma on Indigenous health, the calls for culture to be recognised as central to healing are gathering pace and, in some cases, are finally being heard and acted upon. Here are some examples of successful, culturally-based healing and trauma-informed programs in Australia:

***The Kunga Stopping Violence Program (KSVP)*** is a trauma-informed program for imprisoned Aboriginal and Torres Strait Islander women at the Alice Springs Correctional Centre. Part of the approach includes developing "Loss History Maps", a tool which helps a person tell a life story by identifying significant experiences from birth to the present, allowing them to reflect on how those experiences may be contributing to their present life (ANROWS, 2020, p. 3). An important finding was the difference in resilience levels for those whose childhoods involved being on Country, being taught traditions, and feeling safe in the loving care of grandparents and others who did not drink, and those who grew up in town camps in Alice Springs or Tennant Creek and experienced a lot of family or community fighting fuelled by alcohol (ANROWS, 2020, p. 5).

***TeaH (Turn 'em around Healing)*** is a model of practice that incorporates Aboriginal concepts of healing and spirit within a creative therapeutic framework. It works through principles of community engagement and capacity building, enabling the provision of a culturally-derived intervention that brings together both Aboriginal and Western-based healing practices (Moss & Lee, 2019). Traditional healers in central Australia the*Ngangkaṟi*, explain that "children are born with the spirit that holds itself in culture and language [and] suicide occurs when their spirit is broken" (p. 56). Spirit is thus intrinsic to the *TeaH* model. The authors note in their conclusion that a major public hospital in Adelaide has engaged *Ngangkaṟi* healers to work with their Indigenous patients, making it more likely that Indigenous people will seek medical help when they need it.

***The First 1000 Days Australia model***, based on the international 1000 days movement that calls for action and investment in improving nutrition for the period from a child's conception to their second birthday, was built by adhering to Indigenous methodologies, a recognition of the centrality of culture that reinforces and strengthens families, and uses a holistic view of health and wellbeing. The First 1000 Days Australia was developed under the auspice of Indigenous people's leadership using a collective impact framework. As such, the model emphasises Indigenous leadership, mutual trust and solidarity to achieve early-life equity (Ritte et al., 2016, p. 1).

(*continued*)

**(continued)**

***The Red Dust Healing (RDH) program*** is a cultural healing program written from an Aboriginal and Torres Strait Islander perspective and targeted primarily at Aboriginal and Torres Strait Islander men, women and families (Thompson, 2018). It is used to address a wide range of issues including suicide prevention, Stolen Generations, grief and loss, family and domestic violence, mental health and substance abuse. The program encourages participants to connect with themselves to recognise and confront problems, hurt and anger in their lives, stemming primarily from rejection and grief. The author claims there is "strong evidence of the RDH program positively influencing people's social and emotional wellbeing and that this is often sustained after participation. Respondents report an increased ability to express deep seated emotions, an improved capacity to deal with grief and loss, greater self-awareness and clarity, the ability to make better choices and consequently changes in their lives, increased skills to bring about conflict resolution in the family and community settings and a stronger sense of cultural and spiritual identity" (p. 9).

***A Cultural Healing Program for Aboriginal Survivors of Institutional Child Sexual Abuse*** designed, developed and delivered by an Aboriginal community-controlled organisation, is based on the knowledge that "cultural connection promotes healing, that the collective nature of healing was essential and that healing is a journey" (Black et al., 2019, p. 1066). Cultural connection was achieved by engaging participants in Aboriginal cultural activities and practices and strengthening connections to elders, each other, culture, land and community (Black et al., 2019, p. 1066). The program consists of four sub-programs: a five-day cultural healing camp, a fortnightly women's healing program, a three-day cultural healing gathering and a five-day women's cultural healing gathering. The program design ensured survivors were able to engage in a range of cultural activities and practices that were at times divided into separate men's and women's business. These included ceremonies; cultural practices; a range of arts and crafts; exploring and strengthening identity and connection to community; tracing family history; cultural tours; self-care; healing and wellbeing activities; sharing of knowledge of past policies, laws and history of removal; impact of removal and losses; storytelling and yarning; and sharing of meals (p. 1073).

Feedback from one survivor:

> Cultural healing works, it returns what was taken; this is healing. Strengthening and practicing culture is itself healing. Cultural healing is based on thousands of years of wisdom and the potential power of cultural healing needs to be acknowledged and amplified (Black et al., 2019, p. 1077).

(*continued*)

**(continued)**

***The Healing Centres Project*** is a mission rehabilitation project in Western Australia that emphasises how connection to land, memory and community identity are critical to social and emotional wellbeing and healing for Aboriginal and Torres Strait Islander people (Tiwari et al., 2019). It aims to help Stolen Generations Survivors and their descendants come to terms with the trauma caused by removal policies by establishing Healing Centres at mission sites where they were incarcerated and in which they have direct input in the planning and rehabilitation of these places. The project focuses on two missions where Aboriginal children were taken: Carrolup/Marribank and St Xavier Native Mission at Wandering. "An in-depth contextual understanding of the physical, emotional and ephemeral qualities of the place led to drafting rehabilitation plans that were emotionally and economically sound" (p. 27).

Through dialogue with members of the Carrolup/Marribank and Wandering Survivor community, it became clear that many of the Survivors were still carrying hurt decades after leaving the mission sites. Survivors were at different stages of readiness, many not wanting to visit the site or share their stories with each other, while others were ready to discuss their visions for the sites (p. 31). For the project, the realisation that not all Survivors wanted to achieve the same outcome for the site was a challenge. They all wanted the site to return to its previous condition, but were divided in how they considered the future. Some buildings carried particularly hurtful memories for some, but not for others. Some wanted to promote tourism and others not so much. The project organisers recognise that consultation "will be a long, patient process" (p. 31).

The vision for the project is that traditional cultural practices will influence the process of site development during the building restoration process at Wandering and that Survivors will be involved in physical restoration. This will ensure commencement of a healing process from the very beginning of the project and its continuation throughout the construction and renovation process, especially in the initial stages of the framework.

To conclude, for other examples of promising healing practices for Aboriginal and Torres Strait Islander Peoples see Feeney (2009).

## The 6Rs of Culturally Responsive Practice: The *Damulgurra* Program Model

> We bring ourselves, just as we are—with all our history, experiences and values—to the process of becoming trauma informed. This is the centre. This is our 'being': the way we show up in the world (Cubillo, 2021).

As we bring this book to a close, we invite you to reflect on this Indigenous-led program model (Fig. 9.9) that draws together so many of the elements of cultural safety in trauma-informed practice we have yarned about at each billabong along our journey. This program has been designed and practised on *Larrakia* Country, located in the Darwin region of the Northern Territory. *Dumulgurra* is the *Larakia* word for 'heart'. The program is guided by *Larrakia* Elder Tony Lee and cultural advisor Sabella Kngwarraye Turner from *Arrernte* Country. They each emphasise that the journey of recovery from trauma must start with the heart, which is why heart and land (Country) are placed at the centre.

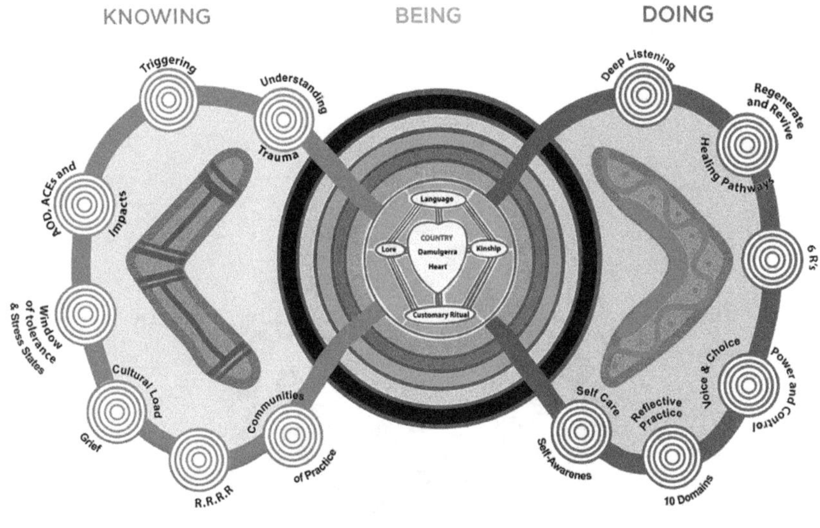


**Fig. 9.9** The *Damulgurra* program model: Knowing, Being and Doing with permission. *Damulgurra* cycles, developed on Larrakia Country for Damulgurra Culturally Responsive Trauma Informed Care, AMSANT. A collaboration between the *Damulgurra* team and *Larrakia* Elder, Tony Lee. Contributors: D. Dyall, A. Jordan, C. Cubillo, K. Randall, J. Smyth and R. Schubert. Artwork by Kyleen Randall

The boomerangs placed inside the two sides of this cyclical process indicate the need to repeatedly reflect on and re-evaluate what we know and how we put that knowledge into practice. Everything is connected, "we can't have knowing without doing or doing without knowing, and all that we know and do will be affected by our sense of 'being'" (Cubillo, 2021).

Notice that this model adds a *6th R* of trauma-informed care: *Regenerate and Revive* (Fig. 9.10).

This is how Carmen Cubillo (2021) describes the 6Rs framework:

> The 6Rs framework acknowledges that we have to *realise* the trauma that has happened to Aboriginal and Torres Strait Islander people, in order to *recognise* the signs and symptoms of trauma. Our aim is to *respond* in a trauma-informed way to *reduce* the ongoing effects of trauma in order to *revive connection* to community, land, culture and ourselves. Our ultimate goal is to empower Aboriginal communities to *regenerate* and *revive* their own local healing frameworks.

We encourage you to learn more about this program, which is one of the strongest examples you could find that reflects an Aboriginal and Torres Strait Islander way of healing from trauma.

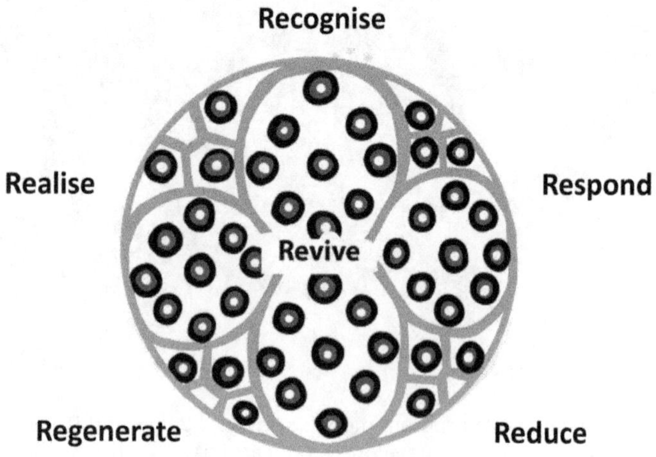


**Fig. 9.10** The 6 Rs. Supplied by Dr Carmen Cubillo with permission

## Concluding Comments

We started our yarn talking about culture. It's a conversation that will always stay alive as there are so many different interpretations and understandings about what culture is. If you think of culture as your roadmap, then it's something that can give you guidance throughout your life. We talked about healing, which involves putting back together the things that have been broken. We also looked at the different knowledge systems we live with in Australia or any country where Indigenous and non-Indigenous cultures exist side by side. We suggested that instead of always privileging one knowledge system, we could start learning more about the intricacies of a knowledge system that kept people alive and thriving for over 60,000 years. While colonisation brought about so much disruption to culture and disconnection of families, it's important to recognise the healing practices that are happening. These include like language rejuvenation, connection to Country, linking up families, yarning and *dadirri,* rituals, and ceremonies still being practised. Reflect on how what this means for you and your work.

**Activity 9.3 Grounding Exercise: Rainstorm**

Like stomping, this exercise is best done in a group. Everyone closes their eyes. Someone starts by making small tapping noises on a book, a table, a desk, sounds that are like rain starting to sprinkle. The next person does the same, mimicking the sound. As you go round the group, everyone just listens to the sound of the gentle rain. Then the person who started makes louder tapping as the rain gets heavier. Others mimic as they go round the room. The sounds become thumps, maybe the feet are involved. It's a big storm now, pouring down on a corrugated iron roof. Then, the storm passes, we hear a few little sprinkles, and then all is quiet. This is an example of a sensory-motor and cognitive grounding exercise.

Reflect in the silence as the storm passes:

- What could you hear?
- What could you feel?
- What was going on for you as you activated your body to make the sounds?
- What part of your brain were you using to listen and to make those sounds?

**Activity 9.4 Check-out and Reflection**

As always, check with what you're feeling and where you feel that in your body after reading this final chapter. Then write responses to the following questions in your journal:

- How would you describe your culture?
- In what ways is your culture a roadmap for your life?
- What would you like to learn more about?
- How could you bring cultural healing into your workplace or practice?

## References and Further Reading

ANROWS (Australia's National Research Organisation for Women's Safety). (2020). *Telling life stories: Exploring the connection between trauma and incarceration for Aboriginal and Torres Strait Islander women.* Retrieved from https://www.anrows.org.au/publication/telling-life-stories-exploring-the-connection-between-trauma-and-incarceration-for-aboriginal-and-torres-strait-islander-women-key-findings-and-future-directions/

Archibald, L. (2006). *Decolonization and healing: Indigenous Experiences in the United States, New Zealand, Australia and Greenland.* Aboriginal Healing Foundation.

Arnold, C., Atchison, J., & McKnight, A. (2021). Reciprocal relationships with trees: rekindling Indigenous wellbeing and identity through the Yuin ontology of oneness. *Australian Geographer, 52*(2), 131–147. https://doi.org/10.1080/00049182.2021.1910111

Barlo, S., Boyd, W. E., Pelizzon, A., & Wilson, S. (2020). Yarning as protected space: Principles and protocols. *AlterNative: An International Journal of Indigenous Peoples, 16*(2), 90–98.

Country, B., Wright, S., Suchet-Pearson, S., Lloyd, K., Burarrwanga, L., Ganambarr, R., Ganambarr-Stubbs, M., Ganambarr, B., & Maymuru, D. (2014). Working with and learning from Country: decentring human authority. *cultural geographies, 22*(2), 269–283. https://doi.org/10.1177/1474474014539248

Berkes, F., Colding, J., & Folke, C. (2008). *Navigating social-ecological systems: Building resilience for complexity and change.* Cambridge University Press.

Bessarab, D., & Ng'andu, B. (2010). Yarning about yarning as a legitimate method in Indigenous research. *International Journal of Critical Indigenous Studies, 3*(1), 37–50.

Bird, R. B., Bird, D. W., Codding, B. F., Parker, C. H., & Jones, J. H. (2008). The "fire stick farming" hypothesis: Australian Aboriginal foraging strategies, biodiversity, and anthropogenic fire mosaics. *Proceedings of the National Academy of Sciences, 105*(39), 14796–14801.

Black, C., Frederico, M., & Bamblett, M. (2019). Healing through connection: an Aboriginal community designed, developed and delivered cultural healing program for Aboriginal survivors of institutional child sexual abuse. *The British Journal of Social Work, 49*(4), 1059–1080. https://doi.org/10.1093/bjsw/bcz059

Blignault, I., Jackson Pulver, L., Fitzpatrick, S., Arkles, R., Williams, M., Haswell, M., & Grand Ortega, M. (2014). *A Resource for Collective Healing for Members of the Stolen Generations: Planning, Implementing and Evaluating Effective Local Responses*. Aboriginal and Torres Strait Islander Healing Foundation.

Burgess, C. P., Johnston, F. H., Berry, H. L., McDonnell, J., Yibarbuk, D., Gunabarra, C., Mileran, A., & Bailie, R. S. (2009). Healthy country, healthy people: The relationship between Indigenous health status and "caring for country". *Medical Journal of Australia, 190*(10), 567–572. https://doi.org/10.5694/j.1326-5377.2009.tb02566.x

Chandler, M. J., & Lalonde, C. (1998). Cultural continuity as a hedge against suicide in Canada's First Nations. *Transcultural Psychiatry, 35*(2), 191–219.

Chandler, M. J., & Lalonde, C. E. (2008). Cultural continuity as a protective factor against suicide in First Nations youth. *Horizons, 10*(1), 68–72.

Corn, A., & Gumbula, N. (2021). *Ancestral precedent as creative inspiration: The influence of Soft Sands on popular song composition in Arnhem Land.* Paper presented at the Power of Knowledge, the Resonance of Tradition Conference, Canberra.

Crouch, K. (2017). Wondering from the womb: antenatal yarning in rural Victoria. *Children Australia, 42*(2), 75–78. https://doi.org/10.1017/cha.2017.15

Cubillo, C. (2021). Trauma-informed care: Culturally responsive practice working with Aboriginal and Torres Strait Islander communities. *InPsych, 43*(3). Retrieved from https://psychology.org.au/for-members/publications/inpsych/2021/august-special-issue-3/trauma-informed-care

Dudgeon, P., Milroy, H., & Walker, R. (2014). *Working together: Aboriginal and Torres Strait Islander mental health and wellbeing principles and practice* (2nd ed.). Commonwealth of Australia.

Enders, G. (2017). *Gut: The inside story of our body's most under-rated organ.* Scribe Publications.

Feeney, M. (2009). *Reclaiming the spirit of well-being: Promising healing practices for Aboriginal and Torres Strait Islander people.* Centre for Applied Psychology, University of Canberra.

Guerin, P., Guerin, B., Tedmanson, D., & Clark, Y. (2011). How can country, spirituality, music and arts contribute to Indigenous mental health and well-being? *Australasian Psychiatry, 19*(1_suppl), S38–S41. https://doi.org/10.3109/10398562.2011.583065

Gooda, M. (2011). One's identity is for the individual to determine. *Sydney Morning Herald.* Retrieved from https://www.smh.com.au/politics/federal/ones-identity-is-for-the-individual-to-determine-20111124-1nwew.html

Grealy, C., Milward, K., & Farmer, J. (2015). *Healing informed organisations: Final report.* Aboriginal & Torres Strait Islander Healing Foundation.

Herman, J. L. (2015). *Trauma and recovery: The aftermath of violence--from domestic abuse to political terror.* Hachette UK.

Hobson, J., Lowe, K., Poetsch, S., & Walsh, M. (Eds.). (2010). *Re-awakening languages: Theory and practice in the revitalisation of Australia's indigenous languages.* Sydney University Press.

Hughes, M., & Barlo, S. (2020). Yarning with country: An indigenist research methodology. *Qualitative Inquiry, 27*(3-4), 353–363. https://doi.org/10.1177/1077800420918889

Jones, R., Thurber, K. A., Chapman, J., D'Este, C., Dunbar, T., Wenitong, M., Lovett, R., et al. (2018). Study protocol: Our cultures count, the Mayi Kuwayu study, a national longitudinal study of Aboriginal and Torres Strait Islander wellbeing. *BMJ Open, 8*(6). https://doi.org/10.1136/bmjopen-2018-023861

Kreutz, G., Murcia, C. Q., & Bongard, S. (2012). Psychoneuroendocrine research on music and health: an overview. In R. MacDonald, G. Kreutz, & L. Mitchell (Eds.), *Music, health and wellbeing* (pp. 457–476). Oxford University Press.

Kwaymullina, A. (2005). Seeing the light: Aboriginal law, learning and sustainable living in country. *Indigenous Law Bulletin, 6*(11), 12–15.

Levine, P. A. (2010). *In an unspoken voice: How the body releases trauma and restores goodness.* North Atlantic Books.

Lou, H. C., Changeux, J.-P., & Rosenstand, A. (2017). Towards a cognitive neuroscience of self-awareness. *Neuroscience & Biobehavioral Reviews, 83*(December), 765–773. https://doi.org/10.1016/j.neubiorev.2016.04.004

Menzies, P. (2008). Developing an Aboriginal healing model for intergenerational trauma. *International Journal of Health Promotion and Education, 46*(2), 41–48. https://doi.org/10.1080/14635240.2008.10708128

Moss, M., & Lee, A. D. (2019). TeaH (Turn 'em around Healing): A therapeutic model for working with traumatised children on Aboriginal communities. *children Australia, 44*(2), 55–59. https://doi.org/10.1017/cha.2019.8

Neale, M., & Kelly, L. (2020). *Songlines: The power and promise.* Thames & Hudson.

Ngaanyatjarra Pitjantjatjara Yankunytjatjara Women's Council Aboriginal Corporation. (2013). *Traditional Healers of Central Australia: Ngangkari.* Magabala Books Aboriginal Corporation.

Pascoe, B. (2014). *Black Emu.* Magabala Books.

Patchett, A. (2021). *These precious days.* Bloomsbury Publishing.

Redvers, N., Yellow Bird, M., Quinn, D., Yunkaporta, T., & Arabena, K. (2020). Molecular decolonization: An Indigenous microcosm perspective of planetary health. *International Journal of Environmental Research and Public Health, 17*(12), 1–13. https://doi.org/10.3390/ijerph17124586

Ritte, R., Panozzo, S., Johnston, L., Agerholm, J., Kvernmo, S. E., Rowley, K., & Arabena, K. (2016). An Australian model of the First 1000 Days: An Indigenous-led process to turn an international initiative into an early-life strategy benefiting indigenous families. *Global Health, Epidemiology and Genomics, 1.* https://doi.org/10.1017/gheg.2016.7

Salzman, M. B. (Ed.). (2018). *A psychology of culture.* Springer International Publishing.

Siegel, D. J. (2012). *The developing mind: How relationships and the brain interact to shape who we are* (2nd ed.). Guildford Press.

The Healing Foundation. (2019). *A theory of change for healing.* Retrieved from https://healingfoundation.org.au/app/uploads/2019/04/HF_Theory_of_Change_A4_Mar2019_WEB.pdf

Thompson, J. (2018). *Red dust healing program: Evaluation.* Caritas Australia & Red Dust Healing.

Tiwari, R., Stephens, J., & Hooper, R. (2019). Mission rehabilitation - A community-centric approach to Aboriginal healing. *Australian Aboriginal Studies, 2*, 19–33.

Ungunmerr, M.-R. (2017). To be listened to in her teaching: Dadirri: Inner deep listening and quiet still awareness. *EarthSong Journal: Perspectives in Ecology, Spirituality and Education, 3*(4), 14–15.

Van der Kolk, B. A. (2015). *The body keeps the score: Brain, mind, and body in the healing of trauma*. Viking Press.

Yunkaporta, T. (2019). *Sand talk: How indigenous thinking can change the world.* Text Publishing.

# Index





N. Tujague, K. Ryan, *Cultural Safety in Trauma-Informed Practice from a First Nations Perspective*, https://doi.org/10.1007/978-3-031-13138-7